T0127699

PLACEMENT LEARNING IN Mental Health Nursing

This book is dedicated to Isaac Stacey

Titles in this series:

Placement Learning in Mental Health Nursing
Gemma Stacey, Anne Felton, Paul Bonham
ISBN 978-0-7020-4303-1

Placement Learning in Medical Nursing
Maggie Maxfield, Michelle Parker
ISBN 978-0-7020-4302-4

Placement Learning in Cancer and Palliative Care Nursing
Penny Howard, Becky Chady
ISBN 978-0-7020-4300-0

Placement Learning in Surgical Nursing
Karen Holland, Michelle Roxburgh
ISBN 978-0-7020-4305-5

Placement Learning in Older People Nursing
Julie McGarry, Philip Clissett, Davina Porock, Wendy Walker
ISBN 978-0-7020-4304-8

Placement Learning in Community Nursing
Jane Harris, Sheila Nimmo
ISBN 978-0-7020-4301-7

Commissioning Editor: Ninette Premdas/Mairi McCubbin
Development Editor: Sally Davies/Carole McMurray
Project Manager: Andrew Riley
Designer/Design Direction: Charles Gray/Miles Hitchen
Illustration Manager: Merlyn Harvey
Illustrator: Graeme Chambers

Placement Learning in

Mental Health
Nursing

A guide for students in practice

Gemma Stacey MN PGCHE RN(Mental Health)
Lecturer in Mental Health and Social Care, School of Nursing, Midwifery and
Physiotherapy, Royal Derby Hospital, Derby, UK

Anne Felton BA(Hons) MN PGCHE RN(Mental Health)
Lecturer in Mental Health and Social Care, School of Nursing, Midwifery and
Physiotherapy, Jubilee Campus, University of Nottingham, Nottingham, UK

Paul Bonham BA MA MEd RMN
Lecturer in Mental Health and Social Care, School of Nursing, Midwifery and
Physiotherapy, Royal Derby Hospital, Derby, UK

Series Editor:
Karen Holland BSc(Hons) MSc CertEd SRN
Research Fellow, School of
Nursing, Midwifery and Social
Work, University of Salford,
Salford, UK

Student Adviser:
Philippa Sharp
Student Nurse, Division of
Nursing, University of
Nottingham, Nottingham, UK

With a contribution from:
Victoria Baldwin MN PGCE RN(Mental Health)
Education and Practice
Consultant, Institute of Mental
Health, Nottingham, UK

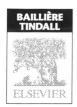

BAILLIÈRE
TINDALL

ELSEVIER

Edinburgh London New York Oxford Philadelphia St Louis Sydney Toronto 2012 'pocket guides' to learning in a range of clinical placements and specific planned placement learning opportunities, and share their content with those who manage this learning experience in practice. We hope that you find them a valued resource and companion during your journey to becoming a qualified nurse.

Karen Holland
Series Editor

Student Foreword

Like most students, I have experienced a range of feelings on starting a new placement: the fears and excitement of what experiences you will have, who you are going to meet and work with, what you will learn, and the responsibilities that come with being that bit further along in your training. These are all feelings that are part of our education and training and contribute to the student's growth as a nurse and as an individual. What is expected of you during a placement is another persistent anxiety, in particular, how you can get the best from that specific placement and how you achieve the gold standard of truly incorporating theory into your practice in an effective and useful way.

Most placement experiences vary in length from introductory 2-week placements to full 18 week hub-and-spoke model placements. It can take a significant amount of the placement time to settle in, understand the way that particular clinical area works and develop an effective professional relationship with your mentor and other members of staff that enables you to learn and achieve.

This series of books makes the gap between what is taught in the University and practiced in clinical placements much smaller and less frightening. It provides guidance on achieving the Nursing and Midwifery Council (NMC) outcomes and competencies, which are essential for becoming a registered nurse, using case studies and real examples to help you. Knowledge of what opportunities to seek in particular clinical areas and how best to achieve them helps considerably, especially when there is so much else to think about. The series also provides a number of opportunities to recap essential knowledge needed for that area (very useful as lectures can seem a long time ago!). For student nurses setting out on that journey to those nearly ending, these books are a valuable resource and support and will help you overcome these sudden panic attacks when you suddenly think 'what do I do now?'. Enjoy them as I have enjoyed being able to have an opportunity to contribute to their development.

Philippa Sharp
3rd Year Student Nurse
University of Nottingham

Introduction

Mental health nursing is an extremely varied and wide-reaching profession. Mental distress is acknowledged as a major health issue in the twenty-first century and is therefore a high priority for every healthcare worker. As a student nurse on placement in a mental healthcare setting, you will have the opportunity to work alongside people who are experiencing mental health problems and accessing mental health services. For some people, their distress is impacting on their quality of life to such an extent that they require additional support. This is often provided by mental health nurses working as part of a team of other professionals such as doctors, occupational therapists and social workers. For some people, the combination of the experience of mental distress, using mental health services and society's perception of mental health problems has excluded them from accessing opportunities to participate in the roles and activities in society that most people would take for granted.

The work of the mental health nurse is stimulating, challenging and dynamic. It requires an appreciation of the impact of social inequalities and injustice to understand a person's distress within their social context. This understanding informs mental health nursing practice and requires the nurse to respond on a psychological, physical and emotional level. The way this might be achieved is not prescriptive and may be influenced by a number of different theories, clinical skills and organisational philosophies. It is also dependent on the individual relationships that are fostered between the nurse and the person requiring support. The nature of these relationships will be influenced by both your own and the person's beliefs, values and attitudes. Commitment to developing an awareness of these and effective interpersonal skills are, therefore, at the core of mental health nursing.

This book aims to facilitate your learning journey in mental health practice settings. It will help you to prepare for your placements by identifying the key areas of learning and offering some practical hints and tips on how to make the most of your placement experiences. It will briefly describe the various areas of service provision and map the care delivery environments you may encounter. It will identify the influential theories, research and policy relevant to contemporary mental health care and help you to identify how these may inform, support or conflict with the practice you are observing and participating in. This will be consolidated through the use of some examples of the varied journeys people could take through mental health services and will encourage you to consider how you could positively impact on their recovery. All case studies and clinical examples given in this book are fictitious in order to protect confidentiality.

The book focuses primarily on approaches and interventions commonly adopted when working with adults with mental health problems. These approaches are also relevant to other age groups, however there are specific interventions which are more widely used with young people and older adults. It is beyond the scope of this book to provide an in-depth discussion of the clinical skills adopted in each of these areas of practice and, therefore, further reading has been recommended should you have a placement which primarily works with these age groups. However, this book will encourage and prompt you to identify how the skills that you are learning on all your mental health placements can be used across different settings.

The book is divided into three main sections:

Section 1: Preparing for practice placement experience

This section will introduce you to the context, history and role of mental health nursing practice. It will identify the policy, legislation, theory and research currently influencing mental health services which will provide you with a core knowledge base in preparation for your mental health placements. It will also give you an outline of mental health placements from the perspective of students, mentors and mental health practitioners. This aims to highlight the key learning opportunities in each area to enable you to plan your learning in order to get the most from each placement experience. To support this, Section 1 also addresses the role of the mentor and how the student–mentor relationship can work to enable effective learning in the practice setting alongside the organisation of practice learning in pre-registration education. Finally, some practical issues relating to mental health placements will be highlighted for you to consider before commencing each placement.

Section 2: Practice-based learning and placement learning opportunities

In this section, and given the variety of different clinical placements you could experience, we have focused on identifying the key skills you will have an opportunity to observe, contribute to, participate in and lead when working with people who experience a variety of mental health problems. This section hopes to enable you to recognise potential learning opportunities available and identify with your mentor what role you can take within the service users' care. These skills range from assessment to care delivery and evaluation, taking into consideration the challenges you may encounter along the way when working with specific mental health problems or client groups. It will also consider your role as a developing leader of care and illustrate how you may begin to foster these skills from the beginning of your nurse education journey.

Section 3: Reflecting on practice learning

This section will demonstrate how to apply the material in previous sections to a series of extended case studies. This will enable you to make the links between the theoretical knowledge and skills that we have identified in Sections 1 and 2 and the practice of mental health nursing. The case studies are based on examples of service users' journeys through mental health services. While these are common examples, each person you meet in practice will have a different experience or outlook and, therefore, may take an alternative path or respond in a dissimilar way to the descriptions we have given here. This is due to the uniqueness of the individual and their mental health problem and often represents what is both challenging and exciting about mental health nursing practice.

Finally, this section will aim to support you to evaluate your own learning and how to deal with challenges you may encounter to improve the quality of your learning experience.

Nursing and Midwifery Council

Before starting to use this book to support your practice learning, it is important to think about how it might link with the outcomes and competencies you are working towards in practice.

As you may be aware from your experiences on your course so far, the Nursing and Midwifery Council (NMC) is nursing's (and midwifery's) regulatory body. This means that it is responsible for setting and monitoring standards of work and conduct for nurses and midwives to maintain. The NMC therefore acts as a means to help safeguard the public by ensuring the health care delivered by nurses and midwives is of high quality.

In order to ensure that nurses are qualifying with the relevant skills and attributes for delivering high standards of person-centred care, the NMC produces standards governing pre-registration education. These outline the skills in which students are required to demonstrate that they are competent in order to progress through their course and ultimately register as a qualified nurse. It is these standards that appear as outcomes or competencies for your mentors to sign off in your record of achievement in practice settings. The NMC (2008) code outlines expectations of conduct and performance for nurses at all times. Compliance with the code is required to maintain safety, high

standards and ensure fitness for practice. The NMC has also produced guidance on professional conduct for nursing and midwifery students (NMC 2009). This code outlines the expectations of conduct, behaviour and performance for student nurses while undertaking their pre-registration education. It can be accessed at http://www.nmc-uk.org/Documents/Guidance/NMC-Guidance-on-professional-conduct-for-nursing-and-midwifery-students.pdf (accessed June 2011).

Chapter 5 highlights how you might be able to use this to prepare for your practice experiences.

NMC standards of proficiency for pre-registration education 2004

Students undertaking training who started their programmes before September 2011 will be working towards the NMC standards of proficiency for pre-registration education (NMC 2004). There are four main domains under which the proficiencies are outlined:
1. Professional and ethical practice.
2. Care delivery.
3. Care management.
4. Personal and professional development.

NMC standards for pre-registration education 2010

There have been a number of changes within healthcare and nurse education. In recognition of the impact this has had on the changing role of the nurse, the NMC updated their standards for pre-registration education to produce new guidelines which were published in 2010. These govern practice learning for anyone who started their pre-registration education from September 2011 onwards.

Here the competencies (term used instead of proficiencies) are outlined under the following four domains:
1. Professional values.

2. Communication and interpersonal skills.
3. Nursing practice and decision making.
4. Leadership, management and team working.

How the NMC proficiencies and competencies relate to Placement Learning in Mental Health Nursing

As you will see as you progress through your placements (and with the support of this book), one activity with an individual using services, their families or other professionals will support you to develop and practise more than one skill, therefore working towards more than one outcome. For instance, writing a care plan with someone will potentially involve proficiencies associated with professional and ethical practice, care delivery, care management and personal and professional development. It is important to bear this in mind when reviewing the chapters in this book.

However, there are some chapters which are more likely to help you with certain domains. This is mapped out in Tables 1 and 2 to help you make the most of

Table 1 NMC proficiencies and related chapters (course start date pre-September 2011)

Domain	Example areas of NMC proficiency (see your practice placement booklets for full outline)	Key chapters
Professional and ethical practice	Awareness of and applying ethical principles to nursing	3
		5
	Awareness of legislation	7
	Maintaining confidentiality	9
		12
Care delivery	Contributing to planning of nursing care	3
	Contributing to implementation of a programme of nursing care	6
		7
	Contributing to identification of potential and actual risks	8
		9
		10
		11
		12
Case management	Demonstrating understanding of the roles of others	2
		13
	Participating in interprofessional working	14
	Demonstrating numeracy, literacy and organising data	6
		9
Personal and professional development	Demonstrating responsibility for own learning and recognising when further learning is required	4
		7
	Demonstrating effective leadership in the establishment and maintenance of safe nursing practice	14
		15
		16

(NMC 2004)

Table 2 NMC competencies and related chapters (course start date post-September 2011)

Domain	Example areas of NMC competency (see your practice placement booklets for full outline)	Key chapters
Professional values	Recognising and addressing ethical challenges relating to people's choices and decision making	3 5 1
	Mental health nurses must practise to address the potential power imbalances between nurses and service users	7 9 13
Communication and interpersonal skills	All nurses must build partnerships and therapeutic relationships	1 3
	Mental health nurses must use skills and knowledge to facilitate therapeutic groups	7 8 6
Nursing practice and decision making	All nurses must use contemporary knowledge and evidence to assess, plan, deliver and evaluate care	2 6 7
	Mental health nurses must be able to apply their knowledge and skills in a range of evidence-based psychological and psychosocial interventions, to assess, develop formulations and negotiate goals	8 9 10 11 12 15
Leadership, management and team working	Nurses must be able to identify priorities and manage time and resources effectively	4 14 15 16

(NMC 2010)

the book. Additionally, many of the activities and reflection points contained in each chapter, once completed, could contribute to evidence for achievement of your proficiencies/competencies and be included in your portfolio. We have signposted these throughout the book, but you may find your own ways of adapting and applying these to provide evidence of your competence, as your experience of placements and developing portfolios builds.

Sources and evidence

In contemporary healthcare contexts, nursing practice should be underpinned by evidence. This is outlined in the NMC standards and many policies that govern mental health care. What is classed as evidence can vary depending on the context. So, in some areas, particularly policy, it relates to published research. However, evidence can also mean clinical experience, expertise and/or other types of literature. This book acknowledges this broad definition of evidence. In developing its content, recent research, service users' perspectives, clinical expertise and students' experiences have been used as evidence to support, develop and challenge the outline of practice learning in mental health placements. Additionally, it highlights the role of a practitioner's (and student's) own values in delivering mental health care alongside these other types of evidence.

References

Nursing and Midwifery Council, 2004. Standards of proficiency for pre-registration nursing education. NMC, London.

Nursing and Midwifery Council, 2008. The code: standards of conduct, performance and ethics for nurses and midwives. NMC, London.

Nursing and Midwifery Council, 2009. Guidance on professional conduct. NMC, London.

Nursing and Midwifery Council, 2010. Standards for pre-registration education. NMC, London.

Acknowledgements

I would like to thank the following students and mentors who have contributed to this book to bring to life the student experience and provide an honest perspective of learning in mental health settings:

Tanya Ames, Gabriella Maria Burton. Charlotte Kawalek, Lucy Mangnall, Polly Murray, Denise Sproat, Sharon Taylor, Ben Thompson, Emily Trivett, Charlotte Turner, Keith Waters, Timothy Westwood, Melissa Wheeler and David Young.

Thanks also to Karen Holland the series editor for providing us with her critical eye and allowing us the flexibility to adapt her concept to a mental health nursing context. Finally, credit goes to my co-authors, contributors and advisers; Anne Felton, Paul Bonham, Victoria Baldwin and Nigel Plant who have enabled this process to be enjoyable and thought provoking.

Gemma Stacey

Section 1. Preparation for practice placement experience

In this section we will focus on what you need to do and learn about before you start a mental health placement for the first time and what to revise if you were returning to different mental health settings.

What's in a name?

Language is a concept that has important implications for people who have used mental health services and mental health professionals. As you progress through the book this will become increasingly apparent as you learn about the importance of being able to develop and sustain hopeful and empowering relationships with people who experience mental health problems and how barriers to this can be created by inequalities in power and prejudice. Within mental health practice and the literature, policy and evidence supporting this practice, you may see people who have direct experience of mental health problems referred to in a number of ways, whether this be as a patient, client, consumer or service user. It is important to highlight that each one of these terms has their specific advantages and disadvantages. There is a lack of agreement among people who experience mental health problems, professionals and policy makers about what the most appropriate language to adopt is. Throughout this book the authors have opted to use the term 'service users' for consistency, and this term also includes people who have experienced mental health problems and people who have used mental health services.

1

Mental health services and nursing: development and practice

CHAPTER AIMS

- To gain an insight into the historical development of mental health services
- To develop an understanding of the role of the mental health nurse in relation to its origins
- To identify activities that a mental health nurse may be involved in and some of the skills used in these activities
- To gain an understanding of the structure of the multidisciplinary team

Introduction

This chapter aims to give an introduction to mental health nursing, locating this in its historical background to help provide a context for some of the key issues in mental health practice. It is constructed to help develop your knowledge of some of the important structures through which mental health care is delivered and the nature of mental health nursing work. This background helps to provide an introductory understanding of what to expect from your mental health placements.

History of mental health services

The history of mental health care and mental health nursing is both a rich and, at times, traumatic one. This discussion is not able to do full justice to the variety of narratives that are integral to this history, nor is it able to give any great depth of detail on the significant events, experiences and policies that make up this history. Yet the importance of understanding history in mental health nursing lies in the significance of the inequalities in power that still exist between nurses and service users. Gaining an insight into where some of these inequalities come from can be helpful in thinking about how they may be bridged. Additionally, through looking back at the history of mental health services, it may aid in appreciating some of the fears and anxieties that someone may have about using mental health services. Ultimately this can help us in delivering care through how we relate to the people in distress that we are working with. Considering the history of mental health nursing also demonstrates how some of the approaches (such as psychological support) have evolved into the interventions used today.

Through a brief description of the key developments of mental health care it is also hoped that you, as a mental health nurse of the future, will be able to gain an appreciation of the past of mental health nursing and the significance of this past in understanding the rewards and challenges of the role in the present.

Institutionalisation

Following the industrial revolution and the relocation of the population in towns and cities, there was a growth in poverty and ill health (Nolan 1993). This represented an increasing problem for those experiencing mental health problems who were unable to afford the private asylums in operation at the time. Within England, concern over the conditions and treatment within private asylums facilitated a drive for lunacy reform (Porter 2002). Subsequent legislation between 1809 and 1845 allowed for the allocation of funds to build public asylums. This reflects a period of the growth of institutions across Europe and Western societies (Wright 1997). It represented a marked optimism for the benefits of the asylum, underpinned by the growing psychiatric profession and the commitment to institutional care as the vehicle to provide a cure for insanity (Rogers & Pilgrim 2001).

Throughout the history of mental health care, the beliefs and understanding of professionals and the public on the causation of mental health problems have influenced the manner in which people have been treated and the drive for "cures". In the early days of asylums, treatments were defined by a need for physical restraint on patients. During this period, in the eighteenth and early nineteenth centuries, individuals caring for the inmates of the asylum were termed 'keepers'. The implications of such a title suggest that those individuals had a role in restricting and controlling the movements of those admitted to the asylum (Nolan 1993).

The optimism for the benefits of a new public asylum system during the mid nineteenth century supported opportunity for the development of pioneering approaches to the management of mental illness developed within the UK and across Europe (Digby 1985, Porter 2002). This included attempts to abandon and reduce the use of physical restraint, examples of which can be seen in the work of Pinel in France, Chiaguri in Italy and Hill and Connelly in England (Porter 2002). 1796 also witnessed the establishment of the York retreat, a Quaker institution founded on the principles of Christian humanism which recognised the humanity of those experiencing mental health problems and promoted moral therapy which attempted to enable individuals to remain included within society (Digby 1985, Nolan 1993).

Within the new public system, after the 1845 Lunacy Act, the role of keeper emerged into one of attendant. The attendant's role was one that involved the most daily contact with people admitted to asylums and they were responsible for their day-to-day care and engagement in work within the asylum. Attendants worked under the direction of the medical superintendent (Nolan 1993). Nolan (1993) notes some early examples of individual superintendents and institutions providing training for attendants but it was not until the very end of the nineteenth century that formalised training was introduced. During this time problems were experienced with the recruitment and conduct of attendants, though pay and conditions were very poor. Pessimism in the asylum system began to spread in the late nineteenth century as asylums became overcrowded and did not deliver the cure for insanity initially hoped for (Porter 2002).

If the history of mental health services and psychiatric hospitals is an area that you are interested in, here is a list of resources that you might find helpful. They include fiction books, video clips and Websites.

FURTHER READING

Faulks, S., 2005. Human traces. Vintage Books, London.

Kesey, K., 1962. One flew over the cuckoo's nest. Penguin, New York.

Kaysen, S., 1993. Girl interrupted. Turtle Books, USA.

WEBSITES

Insights into asylum life:

http://www.countyasylums.com

http://www.highroydshospital.co.uk

State of Mind – series of programmes on BBC Radio 4 examining past and contemporary mental health services:

http://www.bbc.co.uk/radio4/science/stateofmind_20090107.shtml (accessed June 2011)

Podcasts of the Institute of Psychiatry debates on a wide range of topics:

http://www.iop.kcl.ac.uk/podcast/?id=66&type=album

http://studymore.org.uk/mhhtim.htm

 Activity

Once you have accessed one of these resources:

1. Consider one piece of information that has surprised you.
2. What is it about this that was surprising?
3. Identify one issue that you have learnt.
4. What are the implications of this for your practice?

You might want to make a note of some of these issues, in particular the implications for your practice. This can be linked with the activity box on page 21 and included in your portfolio as a record of some of your initial thoughts and reactions at the start of your practice learning journey.

At the turn of the twentieth century, attendants had become known as nurses and the term "mental nurse" was officially instigated on the nursing register in 1923. This reflected the increasing role of psychiatry and the medical approach to understanding mental health problems and therefore nursing was the most appropriate way to care for and treat the mentally ill. During the early part of the century, asylums became known as hospitals. The introduction of the Mental Treatment Act in 1930 represented some attempt to challenge the stigma associated with mental illness that was perpetuated by compulsory treatment through the introduction of voluntary admission. This was underpinned by a desire to treat mental illness within a public health framework (Freeman 1998).

During the twentieth century, further developments in the treatment of mental illness occurred. This included the evolution of a psychodynamic theory pioneered by Freud. However, alongside such developments, treatments were advocated such as psychosurgery which involved removal of parts of the brain thought to be implicated in the symptoms of mental illness. Insulin therapy was also used which involved administering large doses of insulin to cause a coma. These types of treatment, among others, have been heavily criticised as highly dangerous and abusing a population perceived as vulnerable within society. Ion and Beer (2003) warn of the need for us to avoid naively criticising the past without questioning how our own practices may be perceived through the lens of history.

This is particularly poignant given the ethical debates concerning the use of electroconvulsive therapy (ECT) and the damaging impact of psychiatric medication. While there are different perspectives among professionals, service users and families about the use of these interventions today, they are regularly employed to treat mental health problems. The controversies surrounding the use of ECT and psychiatric medication could suggest that their use as treatment may be perceived differently in years to come.

Antipsychotic medication was introduced in the 1950s at a time when the physical state of Victorian asylums was deteriorating and changes in mental health legislation allowed for a more open-door policy within psychiatric hospitals. Public faith in the psychiatric hospital system was diminished through a series of public inquiries and published stories concerning ill treatment, abuse and neglect in hospitals (e.g. Robb 1967). This also occurred within the context of the development of the "antipsychiatry" movement. Key thinkers, such as RD Laing and T Szasz, some of whom were trained psychiatrists, challenged some of the assumptions that mental health problems were a distinct mental illness. A number of antipsychiatrists proposed that mental illness does not exist at all and that people's experiences were the product of an "insane" society. These, combined with other factors, culminated in an announcement by Enoch Powell, in the famous water tower speech, that psychiatric hospitals were consigned to the past and the future of mental healthcare delivery lay in the community. It was also during this time that a humanistic understanding of mental health problems was advocated by Carl Rogers (1967) and the interpersonal nature of nursing was emphasised by the work of Hildegard Peplau (1952).

Over the next 30 years, psychiatric hospitals gradually closed. Historians suggest that care in the community for people with mental health problems has existed for many years including during the asylum era (Wright 1997). However, it is the closure of mental hospitals which contributed to the growth of community nursing and the significant expansion in community services that reflects the model of care delivery we see today. In-patient beds were concentrated in smaller units and district general hospitals rather than distinct large psychiatric hospitals. Many of the service users today who have had long-term needs may have experience of being admitted to an asylum, and this is an area that you might want to explore with them once you have established the therapeutic relationship; particularly considering narratives from people with experience of using services are fairly invisible within the history of mental health care.

This historical overview has given an indication of the negative problems associated with the asylum system which has also been criticised for perpetuating stigma and social exclusion through separating people with mental health problems from the remainder of society.

  Activity

This section has highlighted that closure of asylums contributed to a growth in services delivered in the community and that you may have the opportunity to work with people who have experience of being in hospitals such as these.

Make a list of some of the benefits that people who were admitted there, having all mental health services delivered in the asylum, may have had (the Websites listed above may help you). Also make a list of the disadvantages. Review the list and see how this compares to some of the issues that are highlighted in the section below. You might want to revisit this after your first placement to see whether your views have changed.

However, it is essential to recognise some of the potential benefits of the asylum system, not least as it appeared to offer the best structure for treatment and support to people during their evolution in the Victorian era. Some who have experience of being admitted to psychiatric hospitals speak positively of the peace, quiet and space that were available in the institutions that often had sports grounds, farms and gardens. Social opportunities for connecting with others were also part of the structure of psychiatric hospitals which is important to bear in mind given that isolation remains a barrier to social inclusion and positive mental health for those living in the community.

The majority of mental health services are delivered in the community setting and as a student mental health nurse you will have the opportunity to work in these areas. The evolution of the community teams as the main structures of support for service users provided an important opportunity to challenge the segregation of people with mental health problems and enable people to continue relationships and roles in wider society. This continues to be one of the main areas in which mental health nurses provide support for service users. However, community care has not been without its critics. The closure of psychiatric hospitals and the establishment of community services were chronically underfunded. There was concern that people discharged from psychiatric hospitals were vulnerable to homelessness or ending up as part of the prison population due to a lack of adequate support available in the community setting. During the mid 1990s there were a small number of high-profile incidents of violence related to service users. This led to severe criticism from the press and some charities concerning the appropriateness of supporting people with experience of mental health problems in the community. These incidents and the media and public

response to them have been suggested to have had a significant influence on governmental mental health policy at the time, in particular the development of the Care Programme Approach (Hannigan & Cutcliffe 2002). This is explored in more detail in Chapter 8.

The introduction of *Modernising Mental Health Services* (Department of Health (DH) 1998) and the *National Service Framework for Mental Health* (DH 1999) outlined the hopes of a new government in tackling these concerns regarding the provision of mental health services and for ensuring the care provided to service users was effective and of good quality. These documents had a significant impact on the structure and development of services and were designed to be underpinned by significant financial investment, though there remains concern that the funding imbalances have not been redressed and mental health care remains a "Cinderella service".

Over the past 200 years the role of supporting people with mental health problems has evolved from one of keeper of the insane to one of a mental health nurse working alongside people experiencing mental distress. This overview has provided a very brief insight into some of the factors that have informed and shaped this development. An appreciation of the historical roots of the profession is important in order to understand the issues of power and control experienced within mental health services today. In particular, this concerns the contested nature of treatments in mental health alongside the stigma associated with being "consigned to an institution". Many of these issues bear relevance to today and are picked up in different ways throughout the book. Chapter 3 deals with the philosophies and theories governing contemporary mental health care, some of which you will see have their origins in theories of Rogers and Peplau highlighted here. As you work through this chapter it would be beneficial to think about the similarities and differences between these and what you have read here. Chapter 9 also considers psychiatric medication and enabling people to make choices about their treatment, while Chapter 7 explores the therapeutic relationship and some of the barriers to this. Perhaps more importantly, it is through the professionals and service users that you work with in practice where the relevance of this history may become most apparent, particularly for those who have witnessed and been part of the changes discussed here.

The role of the mental health nurse

What is a mental health nurse?

Mental health nurses work across many diverse settings including GP surgeries, accident and emergency departments, community teams and in-patient psychiatric wards, although there are core skills and values which are integral to this work whatever the setting. This book provides an overview of such capabilities and explores the theory and learning that underpin them in relation to the student practice experience. As you gain familiarity with the literature relating to mental health you may come across debates surrounding the focus and boundaries of the mental health nursing role. This has been influenced by the origin of mental health services, the rapidly changing context of health care over the past 50 years as well as the lack of agreement as to the exact cause and therefore best treatment of mental ill health. This culminates in a situation where it is perhaps more difficult to answer that important question, "what does a mental health nurse do?" than it initially seems.

The last statement has highlighted that it is sometimes difficult to define and identify what is involved in mental health nursing. Often it is a role that can be less visible within media and public information and therefore hard to recognise what it entails until there is the opportunity to gain experience. Some of you may have had this opportunity before starting your first mental health placement.

 Activity

Think about what you believe mental health nursing is. What does it involve?

It might help you to think about the following:

1. What did you say about the role in your application for your nursing course?
2. What did you say during the selection process about what the role of a mental health nurse entailed?
3. How might it differ from previous experiences that you have had (for instance, as a care support worker)?

To follow this up, make a list of eight roles and responsibilities that you perceive that a mental health nurse is involved in. After this, read the following section and move on to the next activity.

Where might a mental health nurse work?

A mental health nurse can work in a vast variety of different settings. Figure 1.1 is an overview of some of the areas where a mental health nurse may work. This provides some examples of the settings where you could be based (though there may be others that you come across in the course of your training). Chapter 5 goes into more specific detail about each of these areas.

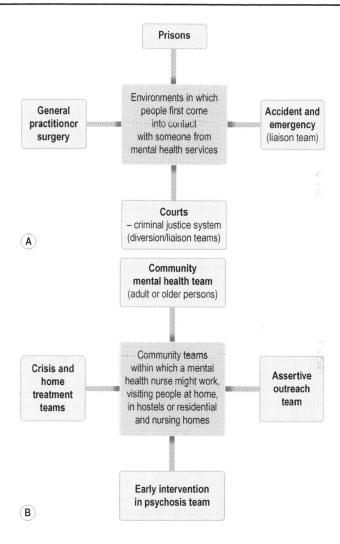

Fig 1.1 Areas of mental health nursing practice. (A) Points of access to service. (B) Community support.

Continued

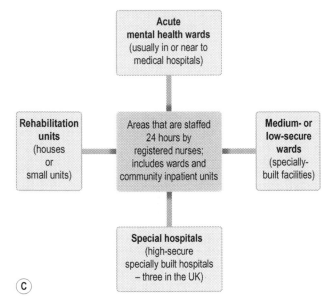

Fig 1.1—cont'd   (C) In-patient care

The following section defines the nature of mental health nursing work in more detail, aiming to help you begin to answer 'so what does a mental health nurse do?'

What does a mental health nurse do?

It is important to recognise that the role of a mental health nurse is not a static one and will be developing and changing in response to new healthcare structures, service user and workforce needs alongside new opportunities. In recent years, these changes have included the introduction of mental health nurse prescribers, nurse consultants and the possibility of nurses being involved in the act of sectioning as approved mental health practitioners (explained in more detail in

Ch. 4). A key nursing theorist, Altschul (1972), described therapeutic relationships as the core of mental health nursing. In this respect the main tool that the mental health nurse has at his or her disposal to impact positively on an individual's health is his or her self. The relationship that a nurse and service user establish is, therefore, central. This means that communicating effectively and learning to really listen and understand another is one of the most important aspects of being a mental health nurse. Without this, the support a nurse is able to provide is limited.

The contemporary mental health nursing role is a complex one. Mental health nurses are involved in working directly with individuals and families to provide support and deal with the impact of being diagnosed with a mental health problem. They will be involved in promoting the health of the individual, but also increasingly working with schools, colleges and communities to promote mental health and enable people to access opportunities outside mental health services to maximise their potential. Mental health nurses are also involved in managing and leading care (examined in Chs 8 and 14) and contributing to the improvement of health care through research and the development and implementation of strategies for enhancing quality.

Through the therapeutic relationship, mental health nurses assess, plan, implement and evaluate care. This is structured through individual time spent with the person.

Assessment

Through interpersonal interaction, sometimes using more formal assessment tools, the mental health nurse will be involved in a process of assessment with the individual experiencing mental distress. This will entail developing an understanding of who it is to be that person at that point in their life (Barker 1997). Integral to this is gaining a holistic perspective which will incorporate an exploration of their mental distress and current problems but also the impact of relationships, social situation, culture, physical health, spirituality and their strengths and coping strategies on their current experiences and future hopes and goals.

Planning care

The nurse will then work with the individual and potentially their family to prioritise the support that they require and develop a plan of care outlining the nature of that support. What this will entail and the resources that it will incorporate will clearly depend on the individual, their experiences and the context in which care is being delivered.

For instance, in an older persons community team (see Ch. 5), a plan may be orientated towards maintaining activities and cognitive stimulation for a person with dementia. Within an in-patient psychiatric ward it may be orientated towards creating a safe environment to enable individuals to explore and manage their distressing experiences. This process is examined in more detail in Section 2.

Outlined below are the areas where a mental health nurse may provide support, followed by some examples of what this might mean.

Support that is provided by a mental health nurse may include the following:
- *Practical:* accessing benefit entitlements or supporting someone with an application for an educational course.
- *Social:* gaining information and helping people to access community resources (such as groups, clubs, courses, gyms) and social opportunities to reduce isolation, extend social networks and enhance self-esteem. It may mean going with them to these activities.
- *Psychological:* exploring the different ways that individuals may cope with hearing voices, helping them to identify what might trigger or make the voices worse and considering different ways of coping that they may not have tried before.
- *Biological:* administering medication alongside outlining support for individuals to regularly monitor their blood sugars for diabetes or plan for supporting an individual who may self-harm with dressing their wounds.
- *Spiritual:* enabling people to access the resources and opportunities that create meaning in their life. This may entail, through the therapeutic relationship, providing a safe space for the person to explore the meaning of their experiences of mental distress.

For the authors, this diversity and breadth of knowledge is integral to building an understanding of individuals in their context. It is also one of the key factors that defines mental health nursing from the other mental health professionals and helps us to be clear about our identity.

The mental health nurse will be engaged in this continual process of assessment, planning, supporting or providing an intervention, evaluating the impact of this and reassessing to inform the next process. This is developed in collaboration with the individual and, where they are involved and consent is given, family and friends. The involvement of the person experiencing mental health problems within this process is essential to ensure that the care provided is meaningful and relevant to them. There are times when this collaboration is challenging, such as when care is enforced through the individual being detained under the Mental Health Act or when a person is so distressed that direct communication about care is difficult. This is a potential tension within mental health services and the role of the mental health nurse.

An introduction to the care programme approach and joint working

One of the main frameworks in the UK, in which this care process is structured in mental health services for adults, is through the Care Programme Approach (CPA). Essentially, this framework was developed to support the increasing amount of care that was delivered in the community in people's own homes. It also aimed to enhance closer working between health and social care services. The CPA sets out the entitlements for the person to have an up-to-date assessment, a care plan that is regularly reviewed and a care coordinator. Mental health nurses are commonly care coordinators although these can also be social workers, psychiatrists and occupational therapists. The role of the care coordinator is to liaise with other professionals to ensure the action in the care plan is being carried out. Mental health services providing care for children and adolescents and older adults (over the

age of 65) follow similar processes although they use different terms for these and are being encouraged by the government to introduce the CPA (DH 2008). Refer to Chapter 9 for more detail about using the CPA.

Paperwork and administration are part of a contemporary mental health nurse's role. They are an important part of communication and working effectively in partnership with others. However, it is difficult to achieve the right balance between the requirements of paperwork and the delivery of direct care. It can be frustrating for a nurse as demands of paperwork feel like they may be getting in the way of direct time with service users. A study by the Sainsbury Centre showed that between 27% and 30% of nurses' time was spent on administration and this was the highest of the mental health professions included (Garcia 2006). They also reported too much time doing paperwork contributed to practitioner stress. It is essential that administration systems are not too complex and bureaucratic leading to high demands on resources being concentrated towards paperwork. It is also important that as practitioners we maintain reflective practice in this area to promote efficient working and help avoid paperwork becoming a barrier to spending quality time with services users.

 Activity

Have a look at the list that you made of the eight roles and responsibilities of the mental health nurse. Consider how this list compares with the outline given above. Is there anything that you would like to add or remove after reading this section?

Keep this list as it will be revisited again in Section 3.

Multidisciplinary team

Within modern healthcare systems, professionals work within multidisciplinary teams. This is perceived as the most effective structure to coordinate the delivery of care and ensures the optimum experience for a service user. Within mental health care, multidisciplinary teams are essential for delivering holistic care which meets the diverse needs and wishes of people with experience of mental distress. It also recognises that the impact of mental health problems can be complex where individuals may benefit from support in a number of areas in their life and that different professionals can offer varied skills and knowledge in these areas.

In response to developing knowledge in mental health care, changing policy and rapidly developing health care, the boundaries of this multidisciplinary team can shift as new roles evolve and change. Figure 1.2 outlines the core roles and professions that you might come across during your mental health placements.

The following discussion considers these roles as they will impact on your experience in placements and the service users you will be working with.

The mental health charity, Mind, have also produced a comprehensive overview of roles in mental health care which can be viewed at: http://www.mind.org.uk/help/research_and_policy/whos_who_in_mental_health_a_brief_guide (accessed June 2011).

Social worker

Social workers tend to be based within community mental health teams. Their background is within the social model (see Ch. 5) and therefore the profession is particularly interested in promoting issues of justice and equality. They have a developing role in relation to personal budgets and direct payments and have played a central role in administering the mental health act.

Occupational therapist

Occupational therapists provide support in areas of occupation. In mental health services this involves assessing and identifying people's interests and capabilities in relation to meaningful activities, often helping people to get access to voluntary work or employment. In some areas this can involve assessing and accessing support aids for activities of daily living within the home environment as well as running social groups. An occupational therapy assistant is an unqualified worker who will provide support for the work of the occupational therapist through direct work with individuals and in groups.

Peer support worker

This is a fairly new role which is rapidly developing. Peer support workers are individuals who themselves have experienced mental distress and provide support to people in a similar situation. Peer support can help people make sense of their experiences and provide inspiration for recovery (Weinstein 2010).

Support time and recovery worker

This role developed with support of the Department of Health to ensure that workers are available with dedicated time to be around service users and provide time and practical support. The introduction of this role promoted an increase in the number of peers employed in this role. Not every team has support time and recovery workers and, in other areas, this role is similar to that of a healthcare assistant.

Psychologist

Clinical psychologists work across different mental health settings. Their focus is on providing psychological support for individuals directed towards their experiences of mental distress and trauma. This tends to be conducted on a one-to-one basis. Psychologists may be involved in delivering different types of psychotherapy

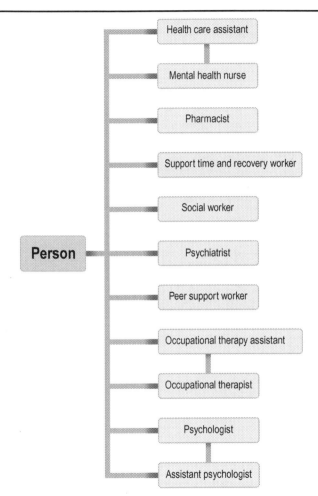

Fig 1.2 Common roles within a mental health multidisciplinary team

such as cognitive behavioural therapy. They may also provide support for service development and facilitate group supervision. Psychology assistants are often individuals gaining an insight into the role prior to undertaking their psychologist training. They will undertake work, with

individuals, who experience mental distress supervised by a psychologist.

Healthcare assistant

Healthcare assistants work closely with the nursing team to provide direct care and support to service users. They most commonly work in in-patient settings though increasingly undertake more autonomous roles in community teams. They are involved in developing relationships with service users and providing practical support. They will often spend the most amount of time with service users and be involved in delivering a plan of care. You may actually have been employed as a healthcare assistant prior to commencing your course, or some of you may be working as a healthcare assistant in non-study time. This can give you some valuable insights into mental health care. However, the importance of knowing the difference between qualified and unqualified will be discussed in Chapter 5.

Psychiatrist

A psychiatrist is a qualified medical practitioner who will have undertaken specialist postgraduate training in order to undertake this role. Most areas will work with a consultant psychiatrist who may have a specialist registrar and more junior doctors as part of their team. Psychiatrists often have overall responsibility for the individuals within their care and have specific knowledge and expertise in relation to diagnosing mental health problems, prescribing psychiatric medication and contribute to decisions regarding compulsory admission to hospital under the Mental Health Act.

Pharmacist

Pharmacists are responsible for preparing medication prior to administration. They have in-depth knowledge relating to the biochemical impact of medication. Pharmacists may be involved in reviewing care with other members of the multidisciplinary team and are able to advise on recommended medications and doses.

Approved mental health practitioner

Prior to amendments to the Mental Health Act (1983), only consultant psychiatrists, GPs and social workers who had undergone specialist training could make the decision that an individual was able to be detained under the Mental Health Act, although mental health nurses, doctors and the police had special holding powers (see Ch. 4). Amendments that were introduced by the government in 2007 extended the professionals that could be approved to conduct assessments and make decisions to detain people in hospital. Currently, social workers, mental health nurses, occupational therapists and psychologists can undertake training to become approved mental health practitioners. This has extended the professionals able to take on a role only previously accessible to social workers. The reaction and acceptance of this role among different professions (including nursing) has been mixed.

Partnership organisations

The complexity of the impact that mental health problems can have on people's lives has already been highlighted. This can mean that input is provided by organisations outside of mental health services. This will clearly depend on the individuals' situation and the nature of their needs. However, it is possible that an individual may be receiving support from general healthcare services, from housing, charitable or advocacy organisations. Some people in distress may need ongoing or intensive input with some of these issues and may therefore live in supported accommodation or hostels provided by such organisations. The changing context of healthcare services suggests that these organisations outside of the NHS, in the voluntary or third sector, are likely to take on an increasing role in providing support across care settings, but in particular to individuals who experience mental health problems or who have learning disabilities (Longley et al 2007). Developing relationships and working in partnership with these organisations is an important area for mental health nurses (explored in more detail in Ch. 15). In this respect, as a mental health nurse you may be working as part of a multidisciplinary and interagency team as well as collaboratively with service users and their loved ones. This contributes to the role of a mental health nurse being a complex yet rewarding one.

 Activity

There will be many opportunities to work with these different professions during your practice experiences. It is likely that you will also meet other students from different disciplines both in practice and theory time. It might be useful to prepare a list of questions that you may have for people from different professional backgrounds, to help you understand their training and role, to aid in future working as part of a multidisciplinary team. Keeping a record of this discussion and reflecting on your responses may contribute to evidence in your portfolio.

References

Altschul, A., 1972. Nurse–patient interaction, a study of interaction patterns in acute psychiatric wards. Churchill Livingstone, Edinburgh.

Barker, P., 1997. Assessment in psychiatric and mental health nursing. Stanley Thornes, Cheltenham.

Department of Health, 1998. Modernising mental health services: safe, sound and supportive. HMSO, London.

Department of Health, 1999. National service framework for mental health, modern standards and service models. HMSO, London.

Department of Health, 2008. Refocusing the care program approach; policy positive practice guidance. HMSO, London.

Digby, A., 1985. Madness, morality and medicine. Cambridge University Press, Cambridge.

Freeman, H., 1998. Mental health policy and practice in the NHS: 1948–79. Journal of Mental Health 7 (3), 225–239.

Garcia, I., 2006. A report on the administrative workload of mental health practitioners, amended version. Sainsbury Centre for Mental Health, London.

Hannigan, B., Cutcliffe, J., 2002. Challenging contemporary mental health policy: time to assuage the coercion? Journal of Advanced Nursing 37 (5), 477–484.

Ion, R., Beer, D., 2003. Valuing the past: the importance of an understanding of the history of psychiatry for healthcare professionals, service users and carers. International Journal of Mental Health Nursing 12, 237–242.

Longley, M., Shaw, C., Dolan, G., 2007. Nursing: towards 2015. Alternative scenarios for healthcare, nursing and nurse education in the UK in 2015. Welsh Institute for Health and Social Care, Pontypridd.

Nolan, P., 1993. A history of mental health nursing. Chapman & Hall, London.

Peplau, H.E., 1952. Interpersonal relations in nursing. GP Putnam's Sons, New York.

Porter, R., 2002. Madness, a brief history. Oxford University Press, Oxford.

Robb, B., 1967. Sans everything. Nelson, London.

Rogers, C., 1967. On becoming a person. A therapist's view of psychotherapy. Constable, London.

Rogers, A., Pilgrim, D., 2001. Mental health policy in Britain, 2nd ed. Palgrave, Basingstoke.

Weinstein, J., 2010. Mental health service user involvement and recovery. Jessica Kingsley, London.

Wright, D., 1997. Getting out of the asylum: understanding the confinement of the insane in the nineteenth century. Social History of Medicine 10, 137–155.

Wycroft, N., 2009. Introduction to nursing. Open University Press, Berkshire.

Further reading

Callaghan, P., Waldrock, H. (Eds.), 2006. Oxford handbook of mental health nursing. Oxford University Press, Oxford.

Clarke, V., Walsh, 2009. Fundamentals of mental health nursing. Open University Press, Berkshire.

Nolan, P., 1993. A history of mental health nursing. Chapman and Hall, London.

Websites

Healthcare roles:
http://www.mind.org.uk/help/research_and_policy/whos_who_in_mental_health_a_brief_guide (accessed June 2011).
http://www.nhscareers.nhs.uk/index.shtml (accessed June 2011).

2 Introduction to the nature and impact of mental health problems

CHAPTER AIMS

- To develop an understanding of the rates and prevalence of mental health problems
- To gain an insight into the impact of mental distress
- To identify the broad nature of mental health problems
- To consider the nature of public attitudes towards people diagnosed with a mental health problem

Introduction

The following chapter will provide a background to the context of mental health nursing in contemporary society. It will consider the relevance and impact of mental ill health and explore some of the challenges that people diagnosed as experiencing mental health problems face.

The aim of this chapter is to enable you to understand the significance of mental health problems and mental wellbeing and identify where mental health nurses fit in relation to wider health and social care services. This provides the background for the remaining chapters, enabling you to gain an insight into mental health nursing in contemporary health care and make links with your experiences during mental health placements.

Mental health problems – frequency and impact

Mental health is described by the World Health Organisation (WHO) (2007, p.1) as "a state of well being in which the individual realises his or her abilities, can cope with the normal stresses of life and can work productively and fruitfully to make a contribution to his or her community". Yet the experience of emotional and psychological distress is a fairly common one. The majority of people will be able to identify times in their lives where they have felt overwhelmed by sadness, anxiety or emotional pain. This is important to bear in mind in any consideration of mental health problems as the issue of mental and emotional wellbeing is increasingly one for each individual, community and institution within our society. It also highlights that mental wellbeing and ill health are part of a continuum. This helps to challenge some of the beliefs within wider society that mental distress and the people who experience it are something to be feared, avoided or shunned. It is when these emotional and psychological experiences become so overwhelming as to restrict the extent to which people are able to live their daily lives, when they persist for a length of time or when they might put that person's (or a) life at risk, that people may be diagnosed as experiencing a mental health problem and benefit from support from a mental health service or professional.

Mental health problems are a major health issue for the global community. The WHO estimates that hundreds of millions of people will experience mental health and neurological problems worldwide (WHO 2010). They also suggest that currently these problems account for the second biggest burden of illness after cardiovascular disease (WHO 2005). This highlights that mental health problems account for a significant health need and are an important area where health and social care services may impact positively on people's lives.

It is important to bear in mind that there are always problems with the measurement of such statistics, as methods of diagnosis may differ and there may be many people in this situation who have not had support from health services. This could mean that some rates may be underestimated. Also a change in attitudes and acceptance towards some experiences may result in individuals being more likely to report this. The following section provides an overview of some of the rates of mental health problems and the implications for healthcare delivery.

International perspective

- An estimated 100 million people in Europe are believed to experience anxiety or depression (WHO 2005).
- 21 million people in Europe are estimated to suffer from alcohol misuse.
- Approximately 4 million people in Europe are estimated to be diagnosed with schizophrenia.

These figures are based on a total population of 870 million (WHO 2005).
- Almost half (45%) of Australians aged between 16 and 85 had experienced at least one mental health problem in their lifetime (Australian Bureau of Statistics 2009).

Common mental health problems

There is evidence to suggest that common mental health problems are increasing in the UK (National Health Service (NHS) Centre for Information 2009a). Common mental health problems are generally those which bring the individual into contact with their GP and will include diagnoses such as depression, anxiety and phobias. Outlined below are some key trends emerging in relation to the changing picture of common mental health problems.
- Around one in six adults are thought to experience mental health problems at any one time (Office for National Statistics (ONS) 2001).
- In England, men are less likely than women to experience a common mental health problem.
- The proportion of the English population who could be diagnosed with a common mental health problem has increased from 15.5% in 1993 to 17.6% in 2007 (NHS Centre for Information 2009a).
- Research suggests that about half of people experiencing common mental health problems are not affected after 18 months, though there is a social inequality in this impact. Those who have long-term sickness due to other conditions, may be unemployed or are of lower socioeconomic status are more likely to still be affected.
- In the Scottish population, between the ages of 15 and 90, the estimated daily use of antidepressant medication has

increased from 1.9% in 1992/1993 to 8.7% in 2005/2006. (Scottish Government 2009).

Serious mental health problems

Serious mental health problems are those which often have a more complex and potentially long-lasting impact on the individual and their lives. This might involve increased support for the person in different areas such as housing, occupation and relationships. This will often involve some periods of care within an in-patient setting. People with serious mental health problems may have experiences such as hearing voices, or have distressing beliefs which are defined as outside the norm. They may have a diagnosis of schizophrenia or bipolar disorder

- People with serious mental health problems have a reduced life expectancy and some evidence has suggested that this is up to 25 years less than the average adult population, a statistic reported in both Europe and America (Parks et al 2006).
- Detentions to hospital under the Mental Health Act in the UK rose to 28 100 in 2008/2009 (NHS Centre for Information 2009b).
- People with serious mental health problems are at increased risk of developing coronary heart disease, diabetes and respiratory disease (Sainsbury Centre for Mental Health 2010a,b).

Once you know where you are going for your mental health placement(s), Chapters 4 and 5 will help introduce you to the preparation for these practice areas. However, this chapter has started to introduce some basic information about the problems and challenges people using these services may face and has drawn on evidence to support this. The activity outlined below will help you build on this in relation to the area you are going to.

Activity

Ask yourself the following question about the placement area:

1. What do you already know about who may be receiving these services?
2. What pieces of information from this chapter do you think are most relevant for this?

Then it will be important to identify what other sources might be useful for finding out this information. Below is a list of some possible Websites to access:

- http://www.mind.org.uk
- http://www.mentalhealth.org.uk
- http://www.alzheimers.org.uk
- http://www.rethink.org

When accessing these, find out about the organisation and think about what implications you think there may be for any biases or the reliability of evidence. Keep any notes you make in the introduction to your portfolio. You could draw on these when developing your evidence for your competencies to help you make links between the evidence base and your practice.

Suicide and self-harm

Self-harm can be used as a coping strategy to deal with emotional and psychological distress and may be used by people regardless of a diagnosis of mental health problems. However, considering people who have contact with mental health services have often experienced traumatic lives and are struggling with emotional distress, self-harm is an area where mental health nurses may offer individuals support. Self-harm is considered as a need to inflict physical wounds onto one's own body to deal with severe and often unbearable psychological pain; the harm itself may be an attempt to cope with this and provide an emotional release. This is without intent to commit suicide (Sutton 2007). Self-harm has been described by survivors as a 'painful but understandable' response to distress, a form of silent scream (Pembroke 1994).

- In England, the percentage of people reporting self-harming during their lifetime has increased and the biggest increase has been in young women (16– 24 years old) (NHS Centre for Information 2009a).
- The UK has one of the highest rates of self-harm in Europe (Mental Health Foundation 2006).
- According to reports by parents, 1.3% of 5–10-year-olds have tried to hurt, harm or kill themselves (Meltzer et al 1999).

Suicide is a traumatic and devastating occurrence. However, individuals who may be having suicidal thoughts will still have a need to be valued, understood and listened to (Noonan 2009). There are particular groups who are more at risk of suicide and this includes people who self-harm.

- In England, 5.6% of people aged 16 and over had reported having made a suicide attempt (NHS Centre for Information 2009a) and there is also evidence that in this group there is an increase in reporting of suicidal thoughts.
- After rising for 25 years, the suicide rate in young men fell in the UK between 1998 and 2007 though overall the suicide rate increased in 2008 (ONS 2010).
- Suicide is more common in men in all age groups and is the most common cause of death in men under 35 (Department of Health (DH) 2002).

Substance misuse

Defining problems around substance misuse and dependence can be problematic. Dependence may be physical or

psychological and is generally considered as a need to continue using a substance on a regular and repeated basis (Kipping 2009). Withdrawal or lack of use could lead to experiencing physical or psychological symptoms. Some people may experience mental health problems alongside being dependent on a substance, which is described as dual diagnosis. However, support for people who are dependent on substances also tends to be provided by mental health services.

- The prevalence of alcohol dependency decreased in men between 2000 and 2007 whereas this prevalence stayed the same for women (NHS Information Centre 2009a).
- In the European region, 21 million people are believed to experience alcohol use disorders (WHO 2005).
- 3.4% of adults in England had some indication of being dependent on illicit or illegal drugs. The biggest part of this statistic was for those who were dependent on cannabis only (NHS Information Centre 2009).

Impact of mental health problems

Being diagnosed with a mental health problem will often have an impact on different areas of that person's life. As this section has highlighted, this can include overall wellbeing. Often as a result of society's reactions to the person as well as the barriers they have to overcome, the implications of being diagnosed with a mental health problem can be far reaching. Yet the relationship between mental health problems and these factors is complex. Some are implicated as triggers for mental health problems and social factors are a major contributor to inequalities in health.

Reflection point

Having read the first section of this chapter, make a list of the areas in an individual's life that you think may be impacted by being diagnosed with a mental health problem. Review how this compares to the information outlined below. This is an issue you might want to return to after your first placement, when you have had the opportunity to work with an individual experiencing mental distress. For this person, there may be areas that they identify that you have not thought of or that have not been covered here.

Social impact

- The survey of psychiatric morbidity in England suggested that there was a strong relationship between low household income and experiencing a mental health problem (NHS Information Centre 2009a).
- People with mental health problems are more likely to be separated, divorced or widowed and be living on their own. The relationship between these issues and mental health is complex as they have implications for both contributing to and being an impact of being diagnosed with a mental health problem (Australian Bureau of Statistics 2009).

Housing

- One in four tenants with mental health problems are at risk of losing their home due to rent arrears (Office of the Deputy Prime Minister (ODPM) 2004).
- People with mental health problems are more likely to be unhappy with the housing they are living in and it is four

times more common for them to suggest that this has a negative impact on their health (Mind 2007).
- There is a close relationship between mental health and housing. One in five homeless people who have mental health problems believe that these problems contributed to them becoming homeless (Mind 2007).

Employment

- One in six workers will experience stress, anxiety or depression at any one time and they are more at risk of losing their jobs than other workers (Sainsbury Centre for Mental Health 2010a).
- 24% of people with long-term mental health problems are employed. This is a lower number than any other group with disabilities (ODPM 2004).
- Employers have a legal responsibility not to discriminate against anyone with mental health problems, supported by the Disability Discrimination Act.

Mental health across the lifespan

Mental health problems impact on people of all ages. Specific age groups will have different needs in terms of support for their mental health problems and encouragement to maximise their health and wellbeing. Emotional distress is becoming increasingly evident in younger people. As a consequence, promoting emotional wellbeing is becoming a key issue for schools, though specialist mental health services are available for children and young people who need additional support (see Ch. 4). In the context of an ageing population, it is suggested that mental wellbeing in old age will be an increasing challenge for health services (Longley et al 2007).

Children and young people

- 45% of looked-after children (children in care) are thought to experience mental health problems.
- It is believed between 6000 and 17 000 children and young people care for an adult with mental health problems (ODPM 2004).
- Estimates suggest that around 10% of children will experience a mental health problem at any one time (Mental Health Foundation 2006).

Older adults

- 700 000 people in the UK are thought to experience dementia (Alzheimer's Society 2010).
- It is suggested two out of five older people in care homes experience depression and one in five older people experience depression (Mental Health Foundation 2006).
- The proportion of people with dementia doubles for every 5-year age group (Alzheimer's Society 2010).

Physical health

There are a number of inequalities in the rates of physical illness experienced by those with a diagnosis of mental health problems. The reasons for these inequalities are complex and are likely to be influenced by a number of factors such as long-term use of medication, social opportunities and access to healthy lifestyle choices.

- People with mental health problems are at increased risk of conditions such as coronary heart disease and diabetes (White et al 2009).
- People with schizophrenia are more likely to get bowel cancer (Disability Rights Commission 2006).
- Long-term physical health conditions are more likely to lead to mental health problems (ODPM 2004).

Ethnicity

The prevalence of mental health problems and the use of services varies among different ethnic groups in the UK. A number of explanations have been proposed as to the reasons for this, which include the lack of culturally appropriate mental health care, level of stigma associated with the use of mental health services in some communities and racism within the system and society.

- Men from black African, black Caribbean and other black groups are more likely to be detained under the Mental Health Act.
- Irish-born people living in the UK have a higher rate of suicide.
- 6% of all people with mental health problems who completed the "Count Me In" census relating to ethnic minorities' experiences in mental health services reported that their first language wasn't English (Healthcare Commission 2009).
- Rates of admission to hospital were less than the national average for those from Indian, Chinese and white British groups and were the same as the national average for Pakistani and Bangladeshi groups (Healthcare Commission 2009).

Service use and support

Mental health services, like all areas of health care, are rapidly changing to reflect the needs of contemporary society. This has had an impact on the settings in which health care is delivered, the allocation of resources and the roles and numbers of professionals working in these services (see Ch. 3 for an overview of the historical development of services).

- Reflecting changes in service delivery settings, the number of in-patient beds has fallen by around 23% between 1997 and 2007.
- One-third of people with dementia live in a care home while the remaining two-

thirds live in the community and it is estimated that, in the UK, family carers save the authorities up to £6 billion a year in care costs (Alzheimer's Society 2010).

- 79% of people using community mental health services responded positively about the service they had received (NHS Confederation 2009).
- Between 1999 and 2008, the number of mental health nurses increased by 24% (DH 2009).
- 90% of respondents to the Healthcare Commissions' annual staff survey identified that their role makes a difference to people with mental health problems (NHS Confederation 2009).

A brief overview of some of the prevalence and distribution of mental ill health has highlighted that supporting individuals with experience of mental health problems is a key issue within health care and nurses have an important role in delivering this care.

Public attitudes

To develop an understanding of mental health problems, it is integral to consider these experiences in their social and political context. Throughout history certain health conditions such as HIV and AIDS, cancer and epilepsy have received negative attention within wider society. Public education, better understanding and advancing treatments have often been successful in challenging these views. However, being diagnosed with a mental health problem remains an often misunderstood experience in which some people may feel a need to hide it from friends, family and employers for fear of the detrimental stereotypes that may go alongside such a diagnosis. As nurses, we are also members of the public and are therefore exposed to the same influences which can impact on the development of our own values and beliefs. This book explores, and may challenge, some of these

beliefs and values as we encourage you to examine how these can develop, change or be reinforced throughout your practice as a student nurse and beyond.

🔘 Reflection point

What were your views of people with mental health problems before you started on the pre-registration nursing course? You might want to think about what some of your fears and anxieties were about working with people with mental health problems.

How did your friends and family respond when you reached your decision to work in mental health care or when they found out you were undertaking a placement in a mental health setting?

Exploring these views and perceptions is useful to help develop self-awareness and to start to enable us to recognise that, as nurses and members of the public, we may well have developed some stereotypes and prejudices or be close to people who have these views. Additionally, it is an important part of developing as a professional to be open to having these views challenged and reflecting on the potential impact that they may have on nursing practice. This is examined in more detail in Chapter 5.

Public perceptions of mental health problems can have a significant impact on how individuals feel about their health concerns and ultimately themselves. In 1996, the mental health charity and campaigning organisation Mind conducted a survey of the personal experiences of stigma and discrimination of people who had received a diagnosis of mental illness. This survey found the following (Read & Barker 1996):

- 34% of respondents had been dismissed or forced to resign from their jobs.
- 47% had been abused or harassed in public.

- 25% felt they were at risk of attack in their own homes or forced to move due to harassment.
- 50% felt that they had been unfairly treated in general health care.

While the survey may well be perceived as outdated, these statistics serve as a stark reminder of the distressing impact that being diagnosed with a mental health problem can have, outside of the concerns that people may be dealing with in terms of their mental health. This highlights the potential role for the mental health nurse in helping individuals deal with these issues as well as providing education for family, friends, employers and educators to challenge some of the influence of these points of view. The impact that these attitudes can have has been recognised by the government and leading mental health organisations that have supported national campaigns to improve public attitudes. The government has focused on tackling the social impact, that can be associated with being diagnosed with mental health problems, through promoting social inclusion. This includes challenging stigma and discrimination and improving access to educational and employment opportunities.

In recent years a number of surveys have been commissioned, including by the Royal College of Psychiatrists, to examine the perceptions of the public towards mental health problems. These have presented some important findings:

- Positive attitudes towards people with mental health problems have *decreased* since 1994 (ONS 2008).
- Younger people have less tolerant attitudes than older people (ONS 2008) and the most negative perceptions were expressed by 16–19-year-olds (Crisp et al 2005).
- 89% of respondents in 2007 agreed that virtually anyone can become mentally ill (ONS 2008).
- Drug addiction and alcoholism received the highest percentage of negative

perceptions than any other diagnosis (Crisp et al 2005).

There are many influences on the development of attitudes towards mental health problems. However, the media has been suggested to play a significant role in the public's perceptions (Anderson 2003). Media reporting has tended to depict people with mental health problems in a negative light and the association with dangerousness and violence has been strong (Cutcliffe & Hannigan 2001), both in the reporting of adverse events and within fictional stories and films. The development of attitudes is complex; however, having these strong views represented in such a powerful influence within society undoubtedly fuels fear and stereotypes associated with mental health problems. This culminates in a situation in which reactions towards people with mental health problems can be dominated by fear. In order to help engender a more positive, helpful and understanding image of mental health across the media, a number of campaigns have been supporting more accurate media representations.

For some of you, this placement might be your first experience of meeting and working with people with mental health problems (or the first time you have knowingly been in this situation) and therefore you may well share some of these concerns about the potential for danger and violence from the people you are working with. This view is not uncommon especially as we have already acknowledged that, as nurses, we are also members of the public and exposed to similar influences to everyone else. Contact with people with mental health problems is one of the most powerful ways of challenging prejudice and impacting on stereotypes. Chapter 5 deals with concerns that you may have before starting your placement, such as these, in more detail.

Exploring the nature of public perceptions has highlighted that these can have an impact on a person's health, opportunities and experiences in their community. It has also been recognised that as health professionals we are not immune to developing prejudice and stereotypes and that acknowledging and exploring our own views is an important part of developing as a mental health nurse.

This chapter has provided an overview of some of the prevalence and impact of mental health problems. It aids in providing a context for the remainder of the book, supporting your journey through mental health placements.

References

Alzheimer's Society, 2010. Statistics. Online. Available at: http://www .alzheimers.org. uk/site/scripts/documents_info.php? categoryID=200120&documentID=341 (accessed June 2010).

Anderson, M., 2003. One flew over the psychiatric unit: mental illness and the media. Journal of Psychiatric and Mental Health Nursing 10, 297–306.

Australian Bureau of Statistics, 2009. Australian social trends. Online. Available at:http://www.abs.gov.au/AUSSTATS/abs@.nsf/Lookup/4102. 0Main+Features30March%202009 (accessed March 2010).

Crisp, A., Gelder, M., Goddard, E., Meltzer, H., 2005. Stigmatisation of people with mental illnesses: a follow-up study within the Changing Minds campaign of the Royal College of Psychiatrists. World Psychiatry 4 (2), 106–112.

Cutliffe, J., Hannigan, B., 2001. Mass media, "monsters" and mental health clients: the need for increased lobbying. Journal of Psychiatric and Mental Health Nursing 8, 315–321.

Department of Health, 2002. National suicide strategy for England. Department of Health, London.

Department of Health, 2009. New horizons: towards a shared vision for mental health. Consultation. HMSO, London.

Disability Rights Commission, 2006. Equal treatment: closing the gap. Disability Rights Commission, London.

Healthcare Commission, 2009. Count Me In census. Care Quality Commission, London.

Kipping, C., 2009. The person with co-existing mental health and substance misuse problems. In: Norman, I., Ryrie, I. (Eds.), The art and science of mental health nursing. A textbook of principles and practice. 2nd ed. Open University Press, London.

Longley, M., Shaw, C., Dolan, G., 2007. Nursing: towards 2015, alternative scenarios for healthcare, nursing and nurse education in the UK in 2015. Welsh Institute for Health and Social Care, Pontypridd.

Meltzer, H., Harrington, R., Goodman, R., Jenkins, R., 1999. Children who tried to harm, hurt or kill themselves. HMSO, London.

Mental Health Foundation, 2006. Statistics on mental health. Online. Available at: http://www.mentalhealth.org.uk/information/mental-health-overview/statistics/ (accessed March 2010).

Mind, 2007. Housing and mental health. Online. Available at:http://www.mind. org.uk/help/social_factors/housing_and_mental_health#impact (accessed March 2010).

National Health Service Centre for Information, 2009a. Psychiatric morbidity in England 2007. Results of a household survey. National Health Service Centre for Information, London.

National Health Service Centre for Information, 2009b. In-patients formally detained in hospital under the Mental Health Act 1983 and patients subject to community treatment 1998–99–2008–2009. National Health Service Information, London.

National Health Service Confederation, 2009. Fact sheet: key facts and trends in mental health. NHS Confederation, London.

Noonan, I., 2009. Nursing people who self-harm or are suicidal. In: Norman, I., Ryrie, I. (Eds.), The art and science of mental health nursing. A textbook of principles and practice. 2nd ed. Open University Press, London.

Office of the Deputy Prime Minister, 2004. Social exclusion unit: fact sheet. Mental health, families and carers. ODPM, London.

Office for National Statistics, 2001. Psychiatric morbidity among adults living in private households. Online. Available at:http://www.statistics.gov.uk/downloads/theme_health/psychmorb .pdf (accessed June 2011).

Office for National Statistics, 2008. Attitudes to mental illness, research report. ONS, UK.

Office for National Statistics, 2010. Suicide; rates increase in 2008. Online. Available at: http://www.statistics.gov.uk /cci/nugget.asp?id=1092 (accessed June 2010).

Parks, J., Svendsen, D., Singer, P., et al., 2006. Morbidity and mortality in people with serious mental illness. 13th technical report. National Association of State Mental Health Program Directors (USA). Online. Available at:http://www.nasmhpd.org (accessed June 2011).

Pembroke, L.R. (Ed.), 1994. Self harm: perspectives from personal experience. Cresswell M An appreciation. Survivors speak out. Online. Available at:http://www.soteria.freeuk.com/SHPPEPREFACE.htm. (accessed June 2011).

Read, J., Barker, S., 1996. Not just sticks and stones: a survey of stigma, taboos, discrimination experienced by people with mental health problems. Mind, London.

Sainsbury Centre for Mental Health, 2010a. Mental health inequalities: measuring what counts. SCMH, London.

Sainsbury Centre for Mental Health, 2010b. Removing barriers: the facts about mental health and employment. SCMH, London.

Scottish Government, 2009. Health of Scotland's population – mental health. Online. Available at:http://www.scotland.gov.uk/ (accessed June 2011).

Sutton, J., 2007. Healing the hurt within: understand self-injury and self-harm, and heal the emotional wounds. How To Books Ltd, Oxford.

White, J., Gray, R., Jones, M., 2009. The development of the serious mental illness: physical health improvement profile. J. Psychiatr. Ment. Health Nurs. 16, 493–498.

World Health Organisation, 2005. Mental health, facing the challenges: building the solutions. WHO, Copenhagen.

World Health Organisation, 2007. Mental Health: strengthening mental health promotion. fact sheet No. 220. WHO, Geneva.

World Health Organisation, 2010. Mental health. Online. Available at: http://www.who.int/mental_health/en/ (accessed June 2010).

Further reading

MIND, Information, Help and Advice section. Online. Available at: http://www.mind.org.uk.

Office of the Deputy Prime Minister, 2004. Mental health and social exclusion: Social Exclusion Unit report. Online. Available at: http://www.socialinclusion.org.uk/publications/SEU.pdf (accessed June 2011).

Read, J., Barker, S., 1996b. Not just sticks and stones: a survey of stigma, taboos, discrimination experienced by people with mental health problems. Mind, London.

Website

Royal College of Psychiatrists, publications and mental health information. http://www.rcpsych.ac.uk.

3 Principles of contemporary mental health practice

CHAPTER AIMS

- To demonstrate an understanding of how the principles of recovery apply to a mental health context
- To analyse the role of values in influencing the decisions made in mental health practice
- To critically reflect upon your own values base in relation to the attitudes and beliefs which underpin your understanding of the role of a mental health nurse
- To critically discuss how a range of understandings of mental health problems can inform creative approaches to mental health practice
- To describe the relevance of health policy for nursing practice
- To identify key policy drivers for the delivery of mental health care
- To explain the role of the NICE guidelines
- To introduce the relevant mental health law and how this impacts on the role and responsibilities of the nurse

Introduction

This chapter will introduce the key areas of learning which you can engage in while on mental health placements. A range of contemporary theories and debates will be presented which are currently underpinning the direction of mental health service provision internationally. The picture is not straightforward and many students find the complexity of mental health care difficult to unpick. This section will aim to help you make sense of the practice you observe, and become involved in, by providing you with explanations of the theory, language and concepts and philosophies of mental health care. The activities and reflective exercises will help you to apply these concepts to your own practice in order to prepare you and make the most of your mental health placement experience.

The first of these is the concept of recovery in the context of mental health. You might think of recovery as returning to a state of health which is normal for you, or as a cure to your health problems. This way of understanding recovery has been challenged by many service users who see it quite differently. For them, recovery is more about coming to terms with their experiences and finding a way of moving beyond them to achieve a quality of life which is more acceptable to them. This might mean for some people that their mental health problems will continue, but that they will find a way of getting nearer to achieving their goals, despite them. Other people may view their mental health problems as a spiritual experience or as offering them an insight into a deeper awareness of themselves which they value and build upon. In contrast, some people may have been severely disabled or traumatised by their experience of mental health problems. It is therefore important to begin with how the person views their experience and the sense they are making of it. The history, development and impact of what has now become known as the "recovery movement" will be discussed and you will be encouraged to think about how this might influence the approach you adopt in your own clinical practice.

For many students, this conceptualisation of recovery is quite challenging as it contradicts their understanding of the nurses' role. Students often say that they are initially attracted to nursing because they wish to care for people and help to relieve their health problems. Therefore, the idea that people may not "get better" and that they might address their problems with little or no intervention from professional services is a challenge. What is required is a shift in the way nurses see their role so it is less about caring for people to address their problems and more about working with people towards increased independence.

The values you bring to your practice will influence the way you work with people. This is known as values-based practice (VBP) and is the second concept we will introduce in this chapter. VBP provides us with a framework to consider how the varied values we hold can influence the way we reach decisions in mental health practice. It recognises that if we are to truly promote recovery as a therapeutic intention then an awareness of our personal values is essential. This will enable us to be open to discussing and acting upon the values of the

people we are working with to deliver mental health services and those who are receiving them.

The final section of this chapter will introduce the different explanations for causes of mental distress. It will contain discussion of the psychological, social and biological approaches to working with service users. You may already have an idea about what you think might contribute to a person's mental wellbeing and there is valid evidence to support each of the explanations we discuss. What we suggest is that by having an awareness of these approaches you can work with the person to help them come to their own understanding of the element of their recovery.

Recovery-orientated mental health care

History
Recovery has predominantly emerged from the stories of service users and has been discussed by professionals or academics.

Definition
. . . a deeply personal, unique process of changing one's attitudes, values, feelings, goals, skills, and/or roles. It is a way of living a satisfying, hopeful and contributing life even with the limitations caused by illness. Recovery involves the development of new meaning and purpose in one's life as one grows beyond the catastrophic effects of mental illness.
(Anthony 1993)

Components of recovery
- Finding meaning and hope.
- Re-establishing a positive identity.
- Building a meaningful life.
- Taking responsibility and control.
(Anderson et al 2003)

Underpinning principles of recovery
- Recovery is possible for everyone and will mean something different to every individual.
- The continuation or recurrence of symptoms of a mental health problem does not preclude the person from recovering a meaningful and valued life. Therefore, support should focus on the person's whole life and working towards wider goals.
- Recovery is something a person achieves for him or her self and, while it can be supported by professionals, it should not be dependent on professional intervention and can occur without it.
- It is often the effects of prejudice and discrimination that restrict people's opportunities and not the people themselves. This can stem from the consequence of receiving a psychiatric diagnosis which usually has negative associations.
- The starting point of recovery is the individual's experience and facilitating an understanding of what they have been through.
- Recovery does not have an end point but is a continuous journey of growth and adaptation. This may not be a linear journey and it may well involve setbacks.
- Carers, relatives, friends and colleagues are often a part of a person's recovery and they may face the challenges of recovery themselves.

Barriers to recovery
- Prejudice and discrimination, which prevent people who have experienced mental health problems from participating in everyday life. This obstructs people from engaging in roles, activities and relationships which give life its meaning and is often referred to as social exclusion.

- The lack of belief or reluctance that people may have in their own ability to take control and responsibility.
- The attitudes of people who deliver mental health services who may portray a hopeless picture of the person's future. This is often based on a belief that mental health problems will disable the person for the rest of their life and that they will be incapable of achieving their goals.
- The attitude within organisations that maintenance of mental health is good enough and therefore service users should be discouraged from taking risks which may not have a predictable outcome. This is sometimes called defensive practice and can be as a result of professionals' fear of litigation.
- The nature of the mental health problem itself which has a negative influence on people's mood, motivation to change or perception of themselves.

 Activity

1. Make a list of the 10 things that you most value in your life.
2. Do they fit into categories or themes?
3. Would this be different from or similar to people who experience mental health problems? If so, how? Evidence suggests that when service users are asked this question, the following are commonly prioritised:
   – somewhere to live
   – something to do
   – someone to love.
4. How does your list relate to this list?
5. What have been the barriers for you in achieving these things?
6. What do you think might be the barriers for people who experience mental health problems in achieving these things?

Recovery models

Despite the supposition that recovery from mental health problems does not always necessarily require professional intervention, it has been identified that some elements of professional practice can obstruct the person's attempts to move forward in their journey. Therefore a number of models, frameworks and approaches have been developed in order to encourage recovery-orientated practice in mental health care. The principles stated above consistently underpin these models, however the language used and ways in which they are applied are slightly different. You may or may not see one of these models being implemented in your placement area or hear your mentor talk about the approaches supported by the authors cited here. The evidence to support the impact of implementing some of the models on changing ways of working has emerged (e.g. Stevenson et al 2002, Cook et al 2005, Gordon et al 2005, Berger 2006, Lafferty & Davidson 2006). However, it has been recognised that due to the uniqueness of the recovery experience, traditional outcome measures, such as readmission rates and levels of medication use, are too narrow to appreciate the complexity of the process of recovery.

The following will describe three examples of recovery models or approaches which are currently being implemented in mental health practice. There are other examples, however these are the most commonly adopted in the UK.

Social inclusion and recovery: components of a model for mental health practice – Julie Repper and Rachel Perkins

This model emphasises the potential impact mental health services can have on a person's opportunities for recovery. It draws upon personal accounts of people's experiences of using mental health services and identifies that the stigma that results from contact with mental health services, the side effects of some psychotropic medication and disempowering practices which are present within organisational culture can act as barriers to recovery. Repper and Perkins (2003) maintain that significant change is required in the attitudes of professionals and the ways they perceive their role if recovery-orientated mental health services are to become sustainable. This model identifies three interrelated components which are proposed to promote the principles of recovery among mental health professionals. These include: developing hope-inspiring relationships; facilitating adaptation which enables personal understanding and opportunities to take back control; and promoting inclusion by helping people to access the roles, relationships and activities that are important to them.

Tidal Model – Phillip Barker and Poppy Buchanan-Barker

The Tidal Model has been developed by mental health nurses in collaboration with service users. It is a philosophical approach to the discovery of mental health. This means it is a way of thinking about how people might reclaim their personal story, as a first step towards recovering their lives. It is maintained that the Tidal Model is an approach to recovery as opposed to a rigid system or a set of prescribed procedures. You can learn more about the Tidal Model at http://www.tidal-model.com.

The model adopts a number of metaphors which aim to challenge the authority attached to professional language and promote common understanding. It compares life to a *voyage* which will inevitably involve some *storms* and may leave the person feeling that they are *drowning*. People who negatively influence the person's selfhood are described as *pirates* and may include an abuser or the instigator of trauma. In these circumstances a person may need guiding to a *safe haven* where they can repair their ship and regain their *sea legs* in order to re-embark on their *life course*.

The key difference between the Tidal Model and other recovery models is the principle that in order for the person to retain their selfhood during periods of crisis, recovery needs to start as soon as possible and should not wait until the crisis has passed. The model refers to this period as 'the lowest ebb'. This may well require support from others including mental health services due to the challenge of exercising the level of self-exploration which is required to understand experiences during periods of significant distress.

The core values which underpin the Tidal Model are defined in the 'Ten Commandments'. In essence, these include a focus on the person's story. This is captured from the person's perspective and told in their own language. It is not rephrased into a 'patient history' and translated into professional speech. It requires the professional to express a genuine interest in the person's view of their experiences and be willing to learn from their expertise as opposed to completing the exercise because it is a routine requirement. The person may not recognise their expertise in their experience and therefore find it difficult to tell their story. It is essential, therefore, that nurses communicate their belief in the person and value their point of view. This requires one-to-one time and it is maintained that this should be prioritised within organisations as opposed to being viewed as a luxury.

The 'Ten Commandments' recognise that the person's story will contain insights into what has helped them in the past. This could inform the types of evidence-based intervention that you draw upon to inform the way you help the person. This requires nurses to hold their personal view of what is the best way to help the person back and

redefine their approach based on the person's definition of effective approaches to care. The first step in moving forward is seen as a crucial element of the recovery journey as it allows the person to see what can be done now and gives optimism for the future. It is acknowledged that although the person's circumstances may change, personal growth is challenging and will require the person to be aware of the changes that are occurring and influence the direction of their care. Many people may find this challenging, particularly if they have been excluded from decisions which influenced their life in the past. It is, therefore, the professionals' role to support the person to input into decisions and advocate for their view during the decision-making process. This will be aided by adopting a transparent approach to practice which includes documenting interactions together and continuing to adopt language which allows for mutual understanding.

Values-based mental health nursing practice – K Woodbridge and B Fulford

The influence of personal values on the way we practise as nurses has recently gained recognition in mental health care (see Department of Health (DH) 2004, Woodbridge & Fulford 2005, Cooper 2009). This school of thought identifies that the decisions we make and the way we work are not only influenced by research evidence but also by our values. This recognition prompts us to be aware of what influences our response to a particular person, their behaviour and how this might impact the direction of their care.

Definition
Values-based practice (VBP) is the theory and skills base for effective healthcare decision making where different (and hence potentially conflicting) values are in play (Fulford 2004).

Activity

The term 'values' is difficult to define. To help you start to understand this concept, use the thought bubble in Figure 3.1 to identify any words, phrases or terms you link with the term 'values'. We have started you off with some suggestions. Now try and put this into a definition.

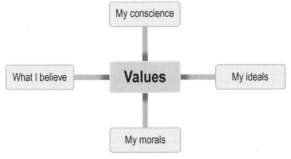

Fig 3.1 What the word 'values' means to me

Values are

....

....

....

....

....

Cooper (2009, p. 22) offers a definition of values: The worth, desirability, importance, or emotional investment (either for or against) we attach to something.

1. How similar or different is this to your definition?
2. What does this tell you about values?

Complexity of values

You may have found that your definition of values is different to Cooper's. This does not mean that it is wrong but it does tell us that values are complex. Woodbridge and Fulford (2003) suggest this is for the following reasons:

Values come in many different varieties

You may have found that your definition is more about ethics, human rights or virtues. Values often encompass all of these things and also go beyond them to take into consideration your own wishes, desires and dreams.

Values vary with time and place and are also eternal

Some values relate to the core beliefs that we tend to think of as with us from childhood and guiding us throughout life. These could be religious beliefs, family values or understanding of what society accepts as right or wrong. However, they can be expressed in different ways or be fluid and changeable depending on life experiences which challenge our values and cause us to question them.

Values vary from person to person

We may have some consensus in what the term 'values' means to us but the individual values we hold may be very different. Also, the importance we place on certain values may be unlike a colleague, service user or friend. For example, you might feel that the value of honesty is highly important to you. However, a colleague may believe that honesty is less important than protecting the person from harm. In this situation you may want to give a person all the information but your colleague may want to withhold it if it could potentially lead to the person becoming distressed.

Values applied to mental health practice

It is important to explore the values that you bring to your work as a student nurse in order to recognise how they are influencing your practice and identify why you may feel in conflict at times with people you are working with. This can include service users, their carers and also your mentor or other professionals. A good way to start this process is by completing the activity in the reflection point box below. This activity will aim to help you clearly define the values you bring to your work. It can become part of your portfolio and you may wish to reflect on it throughout your programme to identify when your values are challenged or reinforced in your practice and how you respond to this.

The values which have been advocated in relation to mental health care were formally brought together in a document called *The Ten Essential Shared Capabilities* (DH 2004). This document was developed in collaboration with service users, carers and mental health practitioners in both the voluntary and statutory sector. It represents a set of overarching principles for the whole of mental health care which aim to promote a recovery-orientated service. These principles were further reinforced in the Chief Nursing Officer's review of mental health nursing which was named *From Values to Action* (DH 2006). This policy sets the direction for the future of mental health nursing practice and emphasises the importance of adopting person-centred values in order to facilitate and promote recovery. A description of these documents and their application is given on Chapter 4.

Principles of values-based practice

Woodbridge and Fulford (2003) have developed the framework of VBP which is defined as:

> . . . the theory and skills base for effective health care decision making where different (and hence potentially conflicting) values are in play.
> (Woodbridge & Fulford 2003, p. 16)

 Reflection point

Developing your nursing philosophy statement (NPS)

A nursing philosophy is a personal statement that describes your own views, beliefs and theories about how nurses should practise and care for service users. There is not necessarily a 'right' or 'wrong' way to write your NPS. However, there are certain issues that you should probably consider when making the connections between what you believe about nursing, how you nurse and how you evaluate your practice.

Most simply, you can start by asking yourself:

1. What are mental health services for?
2. What do you think service users should expect from nursing care?
3. What are your values, attitudes and beliefs about service users?
4. So, what nursing approaches do you use that reflect this position (perhaps with a couple of examples)?

This framework recognises that in order for mental health practitioners to work with values, they should do the following:

- Raise awareness of values. Often, we are not aware of our values until they come into conflict or we feel our values are being ignored. As a professional, our values are usually advocated as a result of the power that is given to us in our role. However, service users often feel their values are dismissed or viewed as less valid as a consequence of their mental health problem. Therefore, it is important to consciously explore values in order to consider how they influence practice. This involves exploring personal values and creating forums for the discussion of values within teams.
- Adopt strategies for reasoning about values which enable the exploration of values which are influencing a situation and justify the outcome of a decision.
- Gain knowledge about the values which are likely to be influencing a situation. For example, gathering the past experiences of people involved, considering how the media may have portrayed a similar situation or exploring research which has been published on the issues arising.
- Adopt communication skills which enable people to give their views and feel listened to. This may involve some negotiation skills or resolution skills where there is conflicting values. This is important in order to ensure that each person's values are given equal attention.
- Start the decision-making process from the perspective of the service user to ensure that practice and policy are applied to the individual.
- Attend to the values of all others involved including the service user's family, friends, informal carers, support workers and all mental health practitioners. This is known as multidisciplinary practice. This will enable potential sources of misunderstanding or conflict to be converted into opportunities for discussion and creative working.
- Consider the influence of both the values and the facts when making decisions. This challenges the assumption that decisions made based on science, such as diagnosis, are not influenced by values of the person conducting the assessment. Values are, in fact, relevant to these decisions and can account for some of the inconsistencies in how different diagnoses are applied to the same symptoms or behaviours.

Barriers to implementing VBP and helpful strategies to facilitate VBP are listed in Table 3.1.

Table 3.1 Barriers and strategies for facilitating VBP

Barriers to implementing VBP	Helpful strategies to facilitate VBP
Forums for the discussion of values are not routinely in place in practice	Clinical supervision, care reviews or multidisciplinary team meetings can be reformatted to enable this discussion
Decisions are sometimes made in an emergency situation which limits the time given to collaboration or effort to involve all parties. Also, when the service user is in crisis,	Crisis planning can allow for people to express their values in anticipation of an emergency situation. Therefore, you can be assured that action taken is in line with a pre-agreed plan. This is where a wellness

Table 3.1 Barriers and strategies for facilitating VBP—cont'd

Barriers to implementing VBP	Helpful strategies to facilitate VBP
they may be seen as unable to contribute to decisions made about their care	recovery action plan (WRAP) or alternative relapse prevention plan can become very useful!
Some people you are working with may not see the value of considering other people's views or be unwilling to listen to alternatives which limits opportunities for negotiation	This will require you to step into their shoes and question why they may find this way of working challenging. The individual may have personal support or professional development needs
The wider organisation of mental health services places the responsibility and accountability of a decision with the professional. This may mean that some professionals are reluctant to consider others' views due to their accountability	A multidisciplinary approach to the decision-making process helps to share this responsibility as it enables concerns to be discussed, explored and strategies to be put in place which the whole team agrees upon. It also allows for the service user to take some responsibility for their actions and feel an increased sense of control

Models of mental health

There are a number of models of mental health which attempt to explain or understand how mental health problems are caused and the ways they are viewed by society. This section will give a brief introduction to the key models which currently influence our understanding and practice in mental health care. What is unusual about mental health problems is that there is no one explanation. Each individual we meet has their own unique experiences, responds to different approaches and has varied journeys through and within their mental health problems. This can be challenging for students and service users because there is no simple explanation or answer. What is important is that the person develops an understanding of their experience which is acceptable to them and therefore the mental health nurses' role often involves supporting them

during the periods of uncertainty, offering possible explanations and helping them to apply this to their own understanding.

Biological

Biological explanations of mental health problems have consistently dominated approaches adopted within mental health services in the UK since psychiatry was first established. This school of thought is sometimes known as the medical model or disease model and views mental health problems as a disease of the brain. It assumes that mental health problems can be assessed and treated in the same way as physical health problems. This involves the identification of a set of symptoms which are grouped together to inform a diagnosis and a plan of treatment. This process is led by a psychiatrist and can require admission to hospital. It often incorporates the use of medication which affects the central nervous system and the ways in which specific neurotransmitters work within the brain. This area of mental health nursing practice will be explored in more detail in Chapter 9.

There are some observable changes in the brain which can influence behaviour. A good example of this is dementia or brain injury resulting from physical trauma. However, the medical model has extended beyond these organic conditions to explain mental health problems such as depression and schizophrenia. These disorders are attributed to factors such as the following:

- A change in the levels of neurotransmitters which can be detected in urine and saliva (Plant & Stephenson 2008).
- Physiological differences such as the size of the temporal lobe in the brain (Gournay 1996).
- A genetic predisposition which is inherited from a family member.

Some people find this approach helpful because it offers them an explanation for their problems and a way of classifying a complex experience. It provides reassurance that others have similar problems and that there are evidence-based treatments which can potentially minimise or eradicate symptoms. However, there are significant criticisms posed at this model of mental health, particularly from service users. These include the following (Norman & Ryrie 2009):

- The assumption that the problem is due to a dysfunction which automatically places the person in a disabled position and therefore at a disadvantage.
- The power that is associated with medical language which can only be understood by those who are educated in the specialist area.
- The tendency for people to become passive recipients of treatment which is prescribed by professionals as opposed to partnerships in their care and recovery.

Psychological

There are a number of schools of thought which fall under the umbrella of psychological models. These include the following.

Psychodynamic

This approach has a primary focus on the ideas and feelings which are behind behaviours, words and actions. It assumes that a significant level of behaviour is determined by mental functioning which we are not aware of. This is influenced by early experiences which occur during childhood and go on to influence the way the person views themselves and the strategies they use to defend themselves as adult. Intervention therefore involves developing an understanding of the different levels of mental functioning known as the conscious and unconscious and addressing negative defence mechanisms.

Cognitive

The cognitive approach is based upon the assumption that the way people interpret their thoughts will subsequently determine their behaviour. The ABC model developed by Ellis (1962) describes this process:

A: activating event.
B: beliefs about the activating event.
C: consequence (emotional or behavioural).

Interventions within this model attempt to identify and alter beliefs about the activating event which are often described as dysfunctional thinking patterns.

Behavioural

The behavioural model is underpinned by learning theory which assumes behaviours are learnt responses that are influenced by external events, stressors and individual personalities. The learnt response is thought to be developed by two key types of conditioning:

1. Classical conditioning (Pavlov 1927)
This term refers to a natural stimulus that becomes associated with an unrelated stimulus response sequence. For example, Pavlov's seminal work illustrated this. In this famous experiment, a dog was conditioned to salivate in response to a bell as opposed to food. Initially the dog was given food at the same time as the sounding of a bell. After a few trials, the dog would salivate at the sound of the bell without the food.

2. Operant conditioning (Skinner 1972)
This results from gaining positive outcome from a behaviour and then applying it to other scenarios (positive reinforcement). For example, Skinner found that rats would initially press levers in a box due to natural curiosity. One of the levers would release food and therefore, after a few tries, the rats learnt to press the lever that released food until they were full, and not to press the other levers.

The behavioural model focuses on changing or replacing a behaviour which is causing the person distress with a more helpful response. This is usually achieved by gradually exposing the person to a stimulus which would normally evoke a negative response and supporting the person to alter how they behave in reaction.

Cognitive and behavioural approaches are often used in combination (cognitive behavioural therapy; CBT). These approaches attempt to address the thinking which underpins a behaviour in combination with changing the behaviour itself. It is recognised that each element can reinforce the other and therefore it is important to address both. This approach is currently gaining increasingly favourable outcomes and has been recommended widely within the National Institute for Health and Clinical Excellence (NICE; 2010) guidelines for a range of mental health problems. Interventions used within this approach will be described in Chapter 11.

Psychological understandings of mental health problems are often positively regarded by service users. They offer the opportunity to build a therapeutic relationship with a professional in order to explore the feelings, thoughts and behaviours which are affecting their mental wellbeing. People often describe feeling genuinely listened to and there appears to be a higher potential for a collaborative working partnership. However, there are limitations to these approaches:

- There is limited evidence which is viewed as 'scientific' to support these approaches due to the many variables that can influence the outcome of the interventions.
- There are often long waiting lists to receive this type of support which limits its accessibility in practice.
- They often require a significant commitment from the individual to the approach. This might include homework, an acceptance that their thinking style or behaviour is problematic and the ability to articulate complex thought and behaviour patterns.
- These requirements are sometimes unrealistic for people who have complex problems and therefore they may be labelled as lacking motivation to change and excluded from psychologically-based therapy on this basis.

Social

The social model focuses on the person in the context of society and considers the influences of social forces on mental wellbeing. Social forces are factors such as isolation, limited relationships, poor living circumstances and unemployment. These factors are suggested to lead to a loss of social role and subsequent alienation from mainstream society which is viewed as the precipitant for mental health problems

(Pilgrim & Rogers 1999). When combined with major life events, such as bereavement and divorce, these factors become even more of an issue because people are not able to draw upon social support or resources to help them cope. Interventions within this model are focused on supporting the person to maintain or re-establish an acceptable role in society through support with employment, relationships and social skills.

According to the social model, all behaviour should be understood from within its social context and the boundary between normal and abnormal should be challenged. The social model is very critical of the medical model because it views the stigma and discrimination which can arise from being given a diagnosis of a mental disorder as significantly damaging to the person's position in society.

The challenges associated with this model are grounded in the difficulties with shifting social beliefs and attitudes in order to challenge social exclusion. This prospect can be extremely overwhelming for the service user and mental health practitioners working in isolation. There has been significant political recognition and investment in strategies to challenge social exclusion for service users. However, research into public attitudes suggests that these interventions have had limited impact on society's core perceptions (Crisp et al 2005).

Integrated approaches

This discussion has briefly outlined the key principles and assumptions associated with the various models of mental health. Each one has advantages and limitations, largely due to their attempts to reduce complex emotional experiences into one explanation. We suggest that each model offers helpful ways of thinking about the possible cause of the person's mental health problems and approaches adopted in mental health nursing are often informed by a combination of each. The approach that

you adopt may be influenced by the philosophy of the organisation or team you are working within, the resources available to you and your own personal values and beliefs about mental health problems. However, we would discourage you from discounting the ideas of a particular model on the basis of personal preference or prejudices. It is helpful to think of these models as the tool box which you can draw upon to inform your practice depending on the individual you are working alongside.

An example of how these models have been brought together is the Stress Vulnerability Model developed by Zubin and Spring (1977). This model is known as a biopsychosocial model. It assumes that we all have a vulnerability to mental health problems, however, for some people, the level of vulnerability is higher. This is as a result of genetic predispositions (biological) and disruptions during childhood (psychodynamic) which can lead to problematic learnt behaviours (behavioural) or a negative perception of self (cognitive). If vulnerability is high, low levels of stress can lead to the experience of mental health problems and major life events are more likely to result in a crisis of mental health. The coping strategies that are employed to deal with stress are suggested to be less well developed due to the impact of negative social circumstances which may have led to poor role modelling or a lack of opportunity to develop supportive social relationships (social). The leaky bucket analogy illustrated in Figure 3.2 can be helpful to explain how each of these factors connect to contribute to a person's vulnerability to mental health problems.

This model continues to be influential in current mental health practice and often informs approaches to working with people who hear voices or have unusual beliefs, such as psychoeducation, relapse prevention and coping skills enhancement. Each of these interventions will be discussed in more detail in Chapter 13.

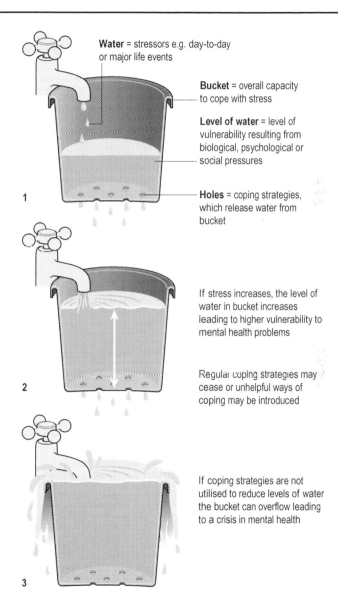

Water = stressors e.g. day-to-day or major life events

Bucket = overall capacity to cope with stress

Level of water = level of vulnerability resulting from biological, psychological or social pressures

Holes = coping strategies, which release water from bucket

1

If stress increases, the level of water in bucket increases leading to higher vulnerability to mental health problems

Regular coping strategies may cease or unhelpful ways of coping may be introduced

2

If coping strategies are not utilised to reduce levels of water the bucket can overflow leading to a crisis in mental health

3

Fig 3.2 The leaky bucket analogy

Mental health policy and law

Policy and law are important areas within mental health care that can impact on the structures and values of service delivery. The following section provides a brief outline of the role of mental health policy and summarises the central mental health policy documents from recent years. While you are a student nurse, it may feel that legal and ethical responsibilities lie with your mentor who is supervising your practice. However, the Nursing and Midwifery Council (NMC) code (2008) states that you are personally accountable for your actions and omissions, regardless of advice or directions from another professional. Therefore, an awareness of the legal frameworks which underpin practice which you are involved in are extremely relevant to you. Furthermore, the mental health nursing skills which are described in this book are underpinned by a requirement to deliver them ethically and in accordance with the law.

Mental health policy

In order to consider the application and relevance of mental health policy in contemporary services, it is useful to briefly explore what is meant by 'policy'. The term is one that to a certain extent defies a definition as there is not a specific agreement about what constitutes policy. However, Lester and Glasby (2006) suggest that policy relates to a series of decisions, acknowledging that those who make the decisions are not necessarily those who will be implementing them into practice. Rogers and Pilgrim (2001) highlight that mental health policy relates to the directives, financial resources and legal frameworks developed for mental health care. They also highlight the sometimes competing functions that this serves in terms of policy being aimed at responding to distress but also controlling behaviour.

Within your practice experiences you will have been directed at some point to the local policies within the organisation where you are working. These local policies provide guidance and direction for specific practices within the local area such as a 'lone worker' policy guiding how to maintain your safety when working in the community. Policy on a national level provides guidelines for the direction of services. This helps to outline and agree the priorities, values and philosophy for care delivery. Certain policies may also be accompanied by financial investment and directives that alter the structure of service delivery. For instance, the *National Service Framework for Mental Health* (DH 1999) supported the development of assertive outreach, early intervention and crisis home treatment teams. This created a path for the services to be delivered nationally.

Table 3.2 contains a summary of some key policies impacting on mental health care.

Table 3.2 Summary of key mental health policy documents

Policy document	Key themes
DH (1999) National service framework for mental health	Developing national standards for health care relating to: mental health promotion, primary care, access to services, care for people with severe mental illness, carers and suicide prevention

Table 3.2 Summary of key mental health policy documents—cont'd

Policy document	Key themes
DH (2001) Journey to recovery; the government's vision for mental health care	Services should support people to work towards recovery. They should work with individuals as partners in their care and be responsive to their needs. These reflect the new government priorities
DH (2002) Women's mental health. into the mainstream. Strategic development of mental health care for women	Highlights that policy, research and services need to recognise the potential differences in the needs of men and women. This includes identifying the need for gender-sensitive and gender-specific services
DH (2004) National service framework for children, young people and maternity services	Focuses on standards for care relating to young people and families. This includes that care provided is person centred and that young people with mental health needs should have an effective assessment. Therapeutic relationships should be developed with young people to promote effective care
DH (2004) National service framework for older people	Outlines set of standards for care relating to older people, including: promoting independence, person-centred care, tackling discrimination. Considers older people and mental health
DH (2004) National suicide prevention strategy for England	Policy to support reduction in suicide through: reducing risk in high-risk groups, mental health promotion and wellbeing, reducing access to methods, promoting research, impact on media reporting and monitoring targets for prevention
DH (2004) Ten essential shared capabilities	Outlines core capabilities for the entire mental health workforce to inform training, continuing professional development and direction of mental health care. Includes focus on: values, social inclusion and recovery, diversity, positive risk taking
DH (2005) Delivering race equality in mental health care; a summary	Recognises inequalities in the care received by black and minority ethnic groups. Outlines action plan to address this through enhancing quality in services and ensuring they are more responsive, that there are better relationships between services and local communities and more effective communication and information sharing
DH (2006) From values to action. Chief Nursing Officer's review of mental health nursing	Provides recommendations for the future direction of mental health nursing in terms of practice and education. This document is centred on recovery and commits to embedding this within training. Also highlights the significance of providing effective support and leadership

Continued

Table 3.2 Summary of key mental health policy documents—cont'd	
Policy document	**Key themes**
DH (2009) New horizons; a shared vision for mental health	The key aims of the policy are to improve the general mental health and wellbeing of the population alongside enhancing the quality and accessibility of support provided to those with poor mental health. This includes recognising need to tackle stigma and discrimination, that mental and physical health care are linked and that there is a need to provide help early

Further details regarding mental health policy may be found at http://www.dh.gov.uk where most of these policies can be downloaded. The approaches to policy across the UK have been similar. For instance, the review of mental health nursing in Scotland was conducted separately and published by the Scottish Executive (2006) but focused on recovery as the driving philosophy for mental health care. However, the structures and impact of these policies may be different within Scotland, Wales and Northern Ireland as each country has legislative powers for policy development in health (Williamson et al 2008). As the publication of mental health policy is linked to national government through the Department of Health, this means the direction of health policy and therefore health services are particularly sensitive to changes in the political views of the ruling government. All of the examples of policy included here were published during a previous government. New health policy will constantly evolve to provide new and a potentially changing direction for health care.

National Institute for Health and Clinical Excellence guidelines

NICE provides national guidelines on the treatment of different health problems. These guidelines are based on a review of the relevant evidence and outline priorities for suggested treatments. They also include an appraisal of the costs and benefits of the interventions, therefore taking into consideration value for money (http://www.nice.org.uk/).

As with any piece of evidence, the NICE guidelines should be viewed critically. It offers evidence-based guidelines that recommend specific standards of practice. However, it has received some criticism for how the evidence it uses is defined. Also some service users and carers feel that some recommendations are driven by cost alone rather than health benefits and quality.

It may be useful for you to read one of these pieces of evidence from NICE prior to your placement, in particular one that relates to the care of the client group in that placement.

 Activity

Using the information from Table 3.2 and any further reading about policy on your next placement:

1. Identify which national policies relate to this placement.
2. Consider the impact that these may have had on practice in that area.
3. Identify some strengths and limitations of these policies on care delivery.

Activity

In preparation for your next placement, identify one of the NICE guideline documents which is relevant to the client group you will be working with. Read the document and consider how this guidance may influence practice. For example:

1. How might it impact on medications which are prescribed?
2. How might it impact on therapies which are offered?
3. How might it impact on the structure of the service and the types of professionals who work within it?

Relevance to practice

Policy has a powerful impact on practice delivery. This is important in terms of working towards national standards, promoting equity of access to care as well as addressing gaps in provision and quality. The start of this section suggested policy is defined as the decision-making process. Recently, there has been a drive towards involving stakeholders in the development of policy, including consultation with professionals and service users, although there have been a number of barriers to these stakeholders having their voices heard, in particular people who have used services (Trivedi 2001). As a mental health nurse, there is an expectation that, beyond initial registration, you will be committed to keeping up to date with changes in evidence and research. This also includes being aware of policy developments and their potential impact on mental health practice.

Given that policy development should include the contribution of key stakeholders such as mental health nurses, there is also a key role for the nurse in shaping as well as responding to mental health policy. This was evidenced in the contribution of mental health professionals as part of the 'Mental Health Alliance' in challenging the government's amendments to the Mental Health Act (see http://www.mentalhealthalliance.org.uk/).

This section has outlined the relevance of policy to mental health practice and linked this to the significant policy documents influencing mental healthcare delivery since 1999.

Mental health law

Law refers to a set of rules or norms of conduct which mandate, prescribe or permit specified relationships among people and organisations. They provide methods for ensuring the fair treatment of people, and provide punishments for those who do not follow the established rules of conduct. The combination of those rules and principles of conduct originate from court decisions and are established by local custom. Practitioners are accountable in law as well as to professional bodies via codes of ethics or conduct.

There are two types of law in England:

1. Common law

This is law made by judges as a result of court cases. There are some very important aspects of health care where practitioners can be held accountable for their behaviour under common law. These include:
- negligence
- confidentiality of personal clinical information
- consent to treatment.

2. Statute law

Acts passed by Parliament. Examples of Acts that set legal standards that the healthcare professional must meet are:
- Mental Health Act 1983/2007
- Human Rights Act 1998
- Data Protection Act 1998
- Mental Capacity Act 2005.

Negligence

Negligence is the breach of a common law duty of care owed to one person by another which results in damage being caused to

---

> ### ⟳ Activity
>
> Legal documents can often be difficult to understand and apply to practice. There are a number of helpful guides which come from reliable sources and help to explain complex law to practitioners and service users. The following links are examples of these:
>
> ■ National Mental Health Development Unit (http://www.nmhdu.org.uk/nmhdu/)
> ■ Mind (http://www.mind.org.uk/)
>
> Use the information provided at these links and the remainder of this chapter to answer the following questions relating to the 2007 Mental Health Act:
>
> 1. What are the key changes to the 1983 Mental Health Act?
> 2. What changes have been made to key roles and responsibilities?
> 3. What are community treatment orders?

that person. Clinical negligence is concerned with claims against doctors, nurses and other healthcare professionals and their employers. In order to succeed in a claim for negligence, the claimant needs to prove the following:

- That the doctor or other healthcare professional owed a duty to take care of the claimant and not cause injury.
- That there was a breach of that duty to take care.
- That the breach of duty has caused harm to the claimant.
- That damage or other losses have resulted from that harm.

For there to be a breach of the duty to take care, it is necessary to show that whatever the healthcare professional, for example the nurse, did or did not do fell below the standard of a reasonably competent nurse in that particular field of health care. This is known as the Bolam Test.

Confidentiality

Service users are legally entitled to expect that information which a healthcare professional learns during the course of clinical practice will remain confidential. The principal legislations concerning the protection and use of personal information are listed below.

- Human Rights Act 1998 – the right to respect for private and family life.
- The Freedom of Information Act 2000 – gives individuals the rights of access to information held by public organisations.
- Data Protection Act 1998 – governs the protection and use of personal information about a living person.
- Mental Capacity Act 2005 – gives individuals who must be involved in decision making on behalf of a person without capacity the right to relevant information.
- The Common Law Duty of Confidence – requires that information that has been provided in confidence may only be used for purposes of which the subject has been informed and given their consent unless there is a legal obligation to disclose. The circumstances making disclosure of confidential information lawful are:
  - where the individual to whom the information relates has consented
  - where disclosure is in the public interest under common law, for example to protect another person from harm
  - where there is a legal duty to do so, for example a court order
  - where an Act of Parliament creates a statutory duty to disclose information.

In the NHS, all healthcare professionals are bound by a legal duty of confidentiality in their contracts of employment and breaching this will lead to disciplinary action and can lead to dismissal. All healthcare professionals are held to an ethical duty of confidentiality by their professional bodies and any breach can lead to disciplinary action. This is stated within *The Code: Standards of Conduct, Performance and Ethics for Nurses and Midwives* (NMC 2008).

Disclosures may be made only in the following circumstances:

- Where they can be justified in the public interest (usually where disclosure is essential to protect the patient or client or someone else from the risk of significant harm).
- Where they are required by law or by order of a court.
- Where there is an issue of child protection.

Reflection point

Think of a time in practice when a disclosure has been made.

1. What contributed to the practitioner making the decision to make the disclosure?
2. What was the impact of this on the people involved?
3. Could the situation have been handled differently to avoid disclosure?

Consent

The ethical principle that each person has a right to self-determination and is entitled to have their autonomy respected finds its expression in law through the notion of consent. For consent to be valid it must be 'real', that is, certain criteria must be met. The service user must:

- have the capacity to give consent
- know in broad terms what they are consenting to

– give their consent freely without being misled, placed under duress or subject to undue influence.

If an adult person meets the criteria to be able to consent to treatment then they also have the right to refuse treatment both at the time it is offered and in the future. Such a refusal of treatment must be respected even if it may lead to the death of the service user. The Mental Health Act 1983 can be used to override a person's competent refusal of treatment for a mental disorder in certain circumstances.

Capacity

Competence is a pivotal concept in decision making about medical treatment. Competent decisions about accepting or rejecting proposed treatment are respected. Incompetent patients' choices, on the other hand, are put to one side, and alternative mechanisms for deciding about their care are sought (Grisso & Applebaum 1998). The legal mechanism for making decisions about the care and treatment of people who lack capacity to make decisions has been governed by statute law since 1 October 2007, due to the Mental Capacity Act 2005.

Statute law

Mental Health Act 1983

This legislation allows service users to be admitted to mental hospitals and detained in appropriate circumstances. Action may only be taken if there is clear evidence that the medical condition of a service user justifies such action. Admission to hospital under the civil sections of the Act (Part II) may only be made where there is a formal application by either an approved mental health professional or the nearest relative. An application is founded on two medical recommendations made by two qualified medical practitioners, one of whom must be approved for the purpose under the Act. Different procedures apply in the case of emergencies.

The most commonly used sections of the Act are the following:
- Section 2 – detention in hospital for assessment for a maximum of 28 days.
- Section 3 – detention in hospital for treatment for up to 6 months which is renewable for a further 6 months and then for 1 year at a time.
- Section 4 – detention in hospital for assessment in cases of emergency for 72 hours maximum.
- Section 5(2) – compulsory detention of informal service users already in hospital for 72 hours.
- Section 5(4) – nurses holding power leading to compulsory detention of informal service users already in hospital for 6 hours.
- Section 17 – leave of absence from hospital: can be given at the order of the responsible clinician (RC), at any time and with any conditions.
- Section 37/41 – detention in hospital which is not time limited. Discharge and leave is restricted by the Home Office as opposed to the resident medical officer.
- Section 58 – treatment which requires consent or a second opinion after 3 months in order to continue. If continued treament is agreed, a form 39 (certificate to treat) is issued.
- Section 117 – under this section, health authorities and local social services authorities have a legal duty to provide aftercare for service users who have been on sections 3, 37, 45a, 47 or 48, but who have left hospital.

Mental Health Act 2007

The Mental Health Act 2007 made changes to the Mental Health Act 1983 through a number of amendments.

Definition of mental disorder

The new Act changes the way in which the 1983 Act defines mental disorder so that a single definition applies throughout the Act and abolishes references to categories of disorder. Section 1(2) states that 'mental disorder' means any disorder or disability of the mind; and 'mentally disordered' shall be construed accordingly. The effect is to widen the application of the provisions in question to all mental disorders.

There is a single exclusion stating that dependence on alcohol or drugs is not to be considered a disorder or disability of the mind for the purposes of the definition of mental disorder.

Appropriate treatment test

This replaced the 'treatable test' and aims to ensure that a service user is only detained if appropriate medical treatment is available to them. However, the definition of medical treatment has also been widened to include psychological intervention and specialist mental health rehabilitation.

Professional roles

The role of responsible clinician (RC) replaces the role of responsible medical officer. The RC could be any professional with the appropriate skills and training. The new legislation also replaces the approved social worker (ASW) with an approved mental health professional (AMHP). The AMHPs will take on the functions of the ASWs and may be suitably skilled and experienced nurses, occupational therapists and psychologists.

Supervised community treatment

The supervised community treatment provisions will allow some service users with mental disorder to live in the community while still being detained under the Mental Health Act. Only those service users who are detained in hospital for treatment will be eligible to be considered and an AMHP needs to be in agreement. Also, to be considered for a community treatment order (CTO), it must be judged that it is necessary for the patient's health or safety or for the protection of other persons that the patient continues to receive their treatment when discharged from hospital. There is a power of recall to hospital for up to 72 hours during which treatment can be imposed under Part IV of the Act. The order lasts initially for 6 months, can be renewed for another 6 months and thereafter for periods of 1 year at a time.

Mental health review tribunals

A maximum period is being introduced during which managers can refer service users to the mental health review tribunal. Managers will be required to refer a service user at 6 months from the day that he/she was first detained and take into account the fact that a patient may have been detained for assessment.

Restricted patients

Section 41 of the Mental Health Act 1983 is amended to remove the power of the Crown Court to make time-limited restriction orders.

Deprivation of liberty

This makes it lawful to detain someone in hospital under the condition that it is an emergency, the person is reliably shown to be suffering from a mental disorder or the disorder is of a nature that warrants compulsory confinement.

Additional safeguards to service users

The new Act gives service users the right to make an application to court to displace their nearest relative and adds the criterion of being 'otherwise not a suitable person to act as such' to the existing criteria for displacement. Civil partnerships will now be recognised as equivalent to marriage under the list of nearest relatives.

The Act also provides the following safeguards:

- Electroconvulsive therapy (ECT) cannot be given to a detained patient who refuses consent except in an emergency situation.
- ECT cannot be given to a person who lacks capacity if it conflicts with an advance decision refusing treatment.

- ECT can only be given to a detained patient under Section 62 when it is immediately necessary to save the patient's life or prevent a serious deterioration in his condition.
- Service users detained under the Mental Health Act 1983 are to be given statutory rights to an advocacy service.
- Trusts must provide age-appropriate accommodation for the treatment of informal and detained service users under the age of 18 with mental health disorders (subject to their needs).

Mental Capacity Act 2005

This Act provides a statutory framework to empower and protect people who lack the capacity to make some decisions for themselves. It generally applies only to people aged 16 or over. It also brings in legal mechanisms that a person with capacity can use to make preparations for a time when they may lack capacity in the future.

The whole Act is underpinned by a set of five key principles set out in Section 1 of the Act:

1. A resumption of capacity – every adult has the right to make his or her own decisions and must be assumed to have capacity to do so unless it is proved otherwise.
2. Individuals being supported to make their own decisions – a person must be given all practicable help before anyone treats them as not being able to make their own decisions.
3. Unwise decisions – just because an individual makes what might be seen as an unwise decision, they should not be treated as lacking capacity to make that decision.
4. Best interests – an act done or decision made under the Act for, or on behalf of, a person who lacks capacity must be done in their best interests.
5. Least restrictive option – anything done for, or on behalf of, a person who lacks

capacity should consider options that are less restrictive of their basic rights and freedoms if they are as effective as the proposed option.

Assessing lack of capacity

The Act sets out a single clear test for assessing whether a person lacks capacity to take a particular decision at a particular time. It is a 'decision-specific' and 'time-specific' test. No one can be labelled 'incapable' simply as a result of a particular medical condition or diagnosis. Section 2 of the Act makes it clear that a lack of capacity cannot be established merely by reference to a person's age, appearance or any condition or aspect of a person's behaviour that might lead others to make unjustified assumptions about capacity. If a doctor or healthcare professional proposes treatment or an examination, they must assess the person's capacity to consent. In settings such as a hospital, this can involve the multidisciplinary team but, ultimately, it is up to the professional responsible for the person's treatment to make sure that capacity has been assessed. A person's capacity must be assessed specifically in terms of their capacity to make a particular decision at the time it needs to be made.

How to assess capacity

Capacity is assessed by asking the following questions:

1. Does the person have an impairment of the mind or brain, or is there some sort of disturbance affecting the way their mind or brain works?
2. If so, does that impairment or disturbance mean that the person is unable to make the decision in question at the time it needs to be made?

A person is unable to make a decision if they cannot:

- understand information about the decision to be made
- retain that information in their mind

- use or weigh that information as part of the decision-making process
- communicate their decision (by talking, using sign language or any other means).

The first three points above need to be applied together. If a person cannot do any of these three things, they will be treated as unable to make the decision. It is sometimes assumed that service users lack capacity as a result of their altered perceptions, unusual beliefs or poor memory.

 Activity

> Consider the following scenario in light of the criteria outlined above.
>
> Brenda is an 87-year-old lady with a diagnosis of early dementia. She is beginning to find it difficult to manage in her home and her children are extremely worried about her safety. Brenda is adamant that she does not want to leave her home and is willing to have help with her day-to-day activities. Brenda's children are not satisfied with this option and are telling your mentor that her mental state is far worse than it appears and that she is not capable of making a decision about her safety.
>
> 1. How might your mentor ascertain if Brenda has capacity to make this decision?
> 2. What factors would influence their decision on Brenda's level of capacity?
> 3. How might your mentor handle the situation to ensure Brenda is safe and the family's worries are calmed?

An act done or decision made for or on behalf of a person who lacks capacity must be in that person's best interests. A person can put his/her wishes and feelings into a written statement if they so wish, which the person making the determination must consider. In addition, people involved in caring for the person lacking capacity have to be consulted concerning a person's best interests.

Acts in connection with care or treatment Section 5 offers statutory protection from liability where a person is performing an act in connection with the care or treatment of someone who lacks capacity. This could cover actions that might otherwise attract criminal prosecution or civil liability if someone has to interfere with the person's body or property in the course of providing care or treatment.

Restraint Section 6 of the Act sets out limitations on Section 5. It defines restraint as the use or threat of force where a person who lacks capacity resists, and any restriction of liberty or movement whether or not the person resists. Restraint is only permitted if the person using it reasonably believes it is necessary to prevent harm to the person who lacks capacity, and if the restraint used is a proportionate response to the likelihood and seriousness of the harm.

Lasting powers of attorney (LPA) The Act allows a person to appoint an attorney to act on their behalf if they should lose capacity in the future. It allows people to empower an attorney to make personal welfare decisions, including healthcare and consent decisions. Before it can be used, an LPA must be registered with the Office of the Public Guardian.

Court-appointed deputies The Act provides for a system of court-appointed deputies who are able to be appointed to take decisions on welfare, healthcare and financial matters as authorised by the Court of Protection but are not able to refuse consent to life-sustaining treatment. They are only appointed if the Court cannot make a one-off decision to resolve the issues.

Court of Protection This court has jurisdiction relating to the whole Act. It has its own procedures and nominated judges. It is able to make declarations, decisions and orders affecting people who lack capacity and make decisions for, or appoint deputies to make decisions on behalf of, people lacking capacity. It deals with decisions concerning property and affairs, as well as health and welfare decisions. It is particularly important in resolving complex or disputed cases involving, for example, whether someone lacks capacity or what action is in their best interests. The court is based in venues in a small number of locations across England and Wales and is supported by a central administration in London.

Public guardian The public guardian has several duties under the Act and is supported in carrying these out by the Office of the Public Guardian. The public guardian and his staff are the registering authority for LPAs and deputies. They supervise deputies appointed by the court and provide information to help the court make decisions. They also work together with other agencies, such as the police and social services, to respond to any concerns raised about the way in which an attorney or deputy is operating. A public guardian board has been appointed to scrutinise and review the way in which the public guardian discharges his functions.

Independent mental capacity advocate (IMCA) An IMCA is someone instructed to support a person who lacks capacity but has no one to speak for him or her, such as family or friends. They have to be involved where decisions are being made about serious medical treatment or a change in the person's accommodation where it is provided or arranged by the NHS or a local authority, and may be involved in abuse cases. The IMCA makes representations about the person's wishes, feelings, beliefs and values and, at the same time, brings to the attention of the decision maker all factors that are relevant to the decision. The IMCA can challenge the decision maker on behalf of the person lacking capacity if necessary.

Advance decisions to refuse treatment The Act creates statutory rules with clear safeguards so that people may make a decision in advance to refuse treatment if they should lack capacity in the future. The Act sets out two important safeguards of validity and applicability in relation to advance decisions. Where an advance decision concerns treatment that is necessary to sustain life, strict formalities must be complied with in order for the advance decision to be applicable. These formalities are that the decision must be in writing, signed and witnessed. In addition, there must be an express statement that the decision stands 'even if life is at risk' which must also be in writing, signed and witnessed.

A criminal offence The Act introduces a new criminal offence of ill treatment or wilful neglect of a person who lacks capacity. A person found guilty of such an offence may be liable to imprisonment for a term of up to 5 years.

The Mental Capacity Act Deprivation of Liberty safeguards The Mental Capacity Act Deprivation of Liberty (MCA DOL) safeguards (formerly known as the Bournewood safeguards) were introduced into the Mental Capacity Act 2005 through the Mental Health Act 2007.

The MCA DOL safeguards apply to anyone:
- aged 18 and over
- who suffers from a mental disorder or disability of the mind, such as dementia or a profound learning disability
- who lacks the capacity to give informed consent to the arrangements made for their care and/or treatment

- for whom deprivation of liberty is considered, after an independent assessment, to be necessary in their best interests to protect them from harm.

The safeguards cover patients in hospitals, and people in care homes registered under the Care Standards Act 2000, whether placed under public or private arrangements. The safeguards are designed to protect the interests of an extremely vulnerable group of service users and to:
- ensure people can be given the care they need in the least restrictive regimes
- prevent arbitrary decisions that deprive vulnerable people of their liberty
- provide safeguards for vulnerable people
- provide them with rights of challenge against unlawful detention
- avoid unnecessary bureaucracy.

Conclusion

The material presented in this chapter is complex and should be considered in preparation for a mental health placement and then reconsidered in light of day-to-day experiences which you have encountered. The scenarios in practice which challenge us often expose the contradictions and dilemmas which exist within ethical and legal frameworks. The answer is rarely obvious and the decision is unlikely to be black or white. The use of clinical judgement is therefore highly important along with the opportunity to discuss and explore with colleagues.

References

Anderson, R., Oades, L., Caputi, P., 2003. The experience of recovery from schizophrenia: toward an empirically validated stage model. Australian and New Zealand Journal of Psychiatry 37, 586–594.

Anthony, W., 1993. Recovery from mental illness: the guiding vision of the mental health service system in the 1990s. Psychosocial Rehabilitation Journal 16, 11–23.

Berger, J.L., 2006. Incorporation of the Tidal Model into the interdisciplinary plan of care – a program quality improvement project. Journal of Psychiatric and Mental Health Nursing 13 (4), 464–467.

Cook, N.R., Phillips, B.N., Sadler, D., 2005. The Tidal Model as experienced by patients and nurses in a regional forensic unit. Journal of Psychiatric and Mental Health Nursing 12 (5), 536–540.

Cooper, L., 2009. Values-based mental health nursing practice. In: Callaghan, P., Playle, J., Cooper, L. (Eds.), Mental health nursing skills. Oxford University Press, Oxford.

Crisp, A., Gelder, M., Goddard, E., Meltzer, H., 2005. Stigmatization of people with mental illness. A follow up study within the Changing Minds campaign of the Royal College of Psychiatrist. World Psychiatry 4 (2), 106–113.

Department of Health, 1999. National service framework for mental health: modern standards and service models. HMSO, London.

Department of Health, 2001. Journey to recovery; the government's vision for mental health care. DH, London.

Department of Health, 2002. Women's mental health: into the mainstream. Strategic development of menatl health care for women. DH, London.

Department of Health, 2004. The ten essential shared capabilities. A framework for the whole of the mental health workforce. DH, London.

Department of Health, 2005. Delivering race equaligy in mental health care; a summary. DH, London.

Department of Health, 2006. From values to action: the Chief Nursing Officer's review of mental health nursing. DH, London.

Department of Health, 2009. New horizons; a shared vision for mental health. DH, London.

Ellis, A., 1962. Reason and emotion in psychiatry. Stuart, New York.

Fulford, K.W.M., 2004. Ten principles of values-based medicine. In: Radden, J. (Ed.), The philosophy of psychiatry: a companion. Oxford University Press, New York.

Gordon, W., Morton, T., Brooks, G., 2005. Launching the Tidal Model: evaluating the evidence. Journal of Psychiatric and Mental Health Nursing 12 (6), 703–712.

Gournay, K., 1996. Schizophrenia: a review of the contemporary literature and implications for mental health nursing theory, practice and education. Journal of Psychiatric and Mental Health Nursing 3, 7–12.

Grisso, T., Appelbaum, P.A., 1998. The assessment of decision-making capacity: a guide for physicians and other health professionals. Oxford University Press, Oxford.

Lafferty, S., Davidson, R., 2006. Person-centred care in practice: an account of the implementation of the Tidal Model in an adult acute admission ward in Glasgow. Mental Health Today (March), 31–34.

Lester, H., Glasby, J., 2006. Mental health policy and practice. Palgrave Macmillan, Basingstoke.

National Institute for Health and Clinical Excellence, 2010. Guidance. NICE, London.

Norman, I., Ryrie, I., 2009. The art and science of mental health nursing. A textbook of principles and practice, 2nd ed. Open University Press, London.

Nursing and Midwifery Council, 2008. The code: standards of conduct, performance and ethics for nurses and midwives. NMC, London.

Pavlov, I., 1927. Conditioned reflexes. Oxford University Press, Oxford.

Pilgrim, D., Rogers, A., 1999. Sociology of mental health and illness. Oxford University Press, Oxford.

Plant, J., Stephenson, J., 2008. Beating stress, anxiety and depression. Piatkus Press, London.

Repper, J., Perkins, R., 2003. Social inclusion and recovery: components of a model for mental health practice. Baillière Tindall, Edinburgh.

Rogers, A., Pilgrim, D., 2001. Mental health policy in Britain, 2nd ed. Palgrave, Basingstoke.

Scottish Executive, 2006. Rights, relationships and recovery: the report of the review of mental health nursing in Scotland. Scottish Executive, Edinburgh.

Skinner, B., 1972. Beyond freedom and dignity, Jonathan Cape, London.

Stevenson, C., Barker, P., Fletcher, E., 2002. Judgement days: developing an evaluation for an innovative nursing model. Journal of Psychiatric and Mental Health Nursing 9, (3), 271–276.

Trivedi, P., 2001. Never again. Openmind 110, 19.

Williamson, G., Jenkinson, T., Proctor-Childs, T., 2008. Contexts of contemporary nursing, second ed. Learning Matters, Exeter.

Woodbridge, K., Fulford, K.W.M., 2003. Good practice? Values-based practice in mental health. Mental Health Practice 7 (2), 30–34.

Woodbridge, K., Fulford, K.W.M., 2005. Whose values? A workbook for values-based practice in mental health care. Sainsbury Centre for Mental Health, London.

Zubin, J., Spring, B., 1977. Vulnerability – A new view of schizophrenia. Journal of Abnormal Psychology 86, 103–126.

Further reading

Barker, P., Buchanan-Barker, P., 2005. The Tidal Model: a guide for mental health professionals. Brunner-Routledge, London and New York.

Brooker, C., Repper, J., 2009. Mental health; from policy to practice. Churchill Livingstone, Edinburgh.

Copeland, M.E., 1997. Wellness recovery action plan. Peach Press, USA.

Lester, H., Glasby, J., 2006. Mental health policy and practice. Palgrave Macmillan, Basingstoke.

Websites

Recovery models:
- WRAP: http://www.mentalhealthrecovery.com
- The Tidal Model: http://www.tidal-model.com

Influential writers in recovery:
- Patricia Deegan: http://www.patdeegan.com
- Rufus May: http://www.rufusmay.com
- Dan Fisher: http://www.power2u.org/who.html

4 Mental health practice learning

CHAPTER AIMS

- To gain an understanding of the nature of various mental health practice areas
- To identify the possible learning opportunities which will enable you to optimise your placement experience and meet your Nursing and Midwifery Council competencies and essential skills clusters
- To consider the views of students and mentors who have experience of working within the practice area
- To develop skills in action planning for placements in order to direct your experience in line with your learning needs

Introduction

This chapter will introduce a variety of mental health placements which you may be given the opportunity to experience as a pre-registration student. The chapter is made up of contributions from students and mentors who have practised in the various clinical areas. The specific name of a service or the way it is structured may vary in your area, however the insights offered by students and practitioners will be helpful in preparing for your placement and getting the most of the learning experience.

Practice learning (placements) may be organised slightly differently depending on the university that you are studying at. These might be in placement blocks of so many weeks in which you rotate around different practice areas with time spent in university during these placements or in between (e.g. one placement in services working with older people, one in a community mental health team and one in an acute in-patient service). Practice learning may have also been organised so that you have a caseload of service users who you follow throughout your training. The changing nature of health care is also facilitating the increasing use of a different structure of practice learning.

The NHS next-stage review outlined a new direction for the configuration of health and social care services promoting increased integration and partnership, requiring health professionals to work across service boundaries (Darzi 2008). In the future, healthcare services will be required to meet a number of challenges including an ageing population, the delivery of care in different environments and rapidly changing technology (Longley et al 2007). In order to help nurses of the

🏴 **Activity**

Have a look through your student handbook alongside your course information and read the sections on practice learning.

1. Identify what approach to practice learning is used in your university.
2. Identify what 'type' of practice settings you might be going to on your course.
3. Consider what you already know about these settings and what you might need to know to help you plan your learning for these areas (Ch. 5 will help you with this).
4. Check the chapter aims and outcomes for Section 2 and highlight the chapters you feel will be most relevant.
5. Write an action plan for how you will find out any further information you need about the practice areas where you will be on placement.

future meet some of the challenges, the Nursing and Midwifery Council (NMC) stipulates that practice learning for students undertaking pre-registration education must reflect the service users' journey in order to support the practitioners of the future to work in reconfigured service structures (NMC 2010).

This means that rather than blocks of placements, universities and the care providers they work in partnership with are increasingly moving towards structuring placements to more closely follow a pathway that a service user may take through services. This might mean that, as a student, you spend longer time working with one mentor, service user or service. One of the important implications of this is identifying how the skills that you are learning can be used effectively in different settings (some of which you might not get

the opportunity to spend lots of time in during your education). This emphasis on how skills can be used in working with individuals in different settings is reflected in the structure of this book, through its focus on approaches and skills important for mental health nursing across service boundaries.

In some courses this pathways approach will mean you are based in one practice area for longer, spending a few weeks during this time in practice areas that link with this service. This might also include shorter insight visits where you may have the opportunity to spend time with different professionals or in settings outside health care (such as the coroner's court). Figure 4.1 shows what this might look like. The centre box represents the main placement area, the lightly shaded boxes may be the practice areas where you could spend a few weeks and the unshaded boxes may be where you link with for insight visits. Depending on your course, this could be arranged for you, or it may be something that you have the opportunity to get involved in arranging yourself following discussion with your mentor.

Routes into mental health services

Mental health support is provided to individuals across the age span in a variety of settings within healthcare services. The manner in which individuals gain access to this support is to a certain extent defined by the nature and priority of their need (in a similar way to access to all health services). However, given some of the tensions that may be associated with mental health care, including care delivered to individuals detained under the Mental Health Act, the means through which initial contact is established could have major implications for the development of the therapeutic

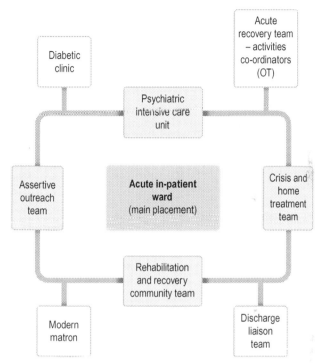

Fig 4.1 Example of a pathway learning experience in mental health

relationship and the delivery of the required support.

GPs remain one of the main gatekeepers to mental health services and, in many respects, GP surgeries are a major provider of mental health support. However, GPs refer to both primary and secondary mental health services (there will be some local variations in the design of these services). Counselling and psychotherapy services are delivered by mental health nurses and specially trained mental health workers in GP surgeries. These practitioners provide support for individuals with common mental health problems or who may be experiencing trauma and can gain

psychological input for their experiences on a short-term basis. GPs will refer directly to these practitioners. They may also refer people on to community mental health teams of which there are a number of different types (see Ch. 6). The circumstances and diagnosis of each individual may define where they are referred. Here, professionals working in the community (commonly mental health nurses) will conduct an assessment to decide whether they are the appropriate people to provide support. For people who are highly distressed and in immediate need, GPs can also refer directly to a crisis and home treatment team. This service can provide short-term and intensive support to the individual in his or her own home until the crisis period is over. They can also work towards securing an admission to hospital for the individual if this is required.

For access to mental health services, support or hospital admission out of hours, the accident and emergency department might be a first port of call which can result in an assessment by a psychiatrist, referral to a crisis team or, in some areas, short-term input from a specialist accident and emergency liaison team.

People can also come into contact with mental health services via the police and the criminal justice system. Mental health services have received criticism due to the inequalities in access among different ethnic groups, as Afro-Caribbean men are more likely to come into contact with mental health services via the police. Rates of mental health problems are high among prisoners and this group is at particularly high risk in relation to suicide. Prison in-reach teams may take on referrals from people in prison experiencing mental distress. At times this can result in individuals who require support being moved to forensic secure units or hospitals. If an individual is arrested and there is concern they may have mental health problems, forensic or court liaison teams may conduct assessments to identify whether the person requires the input of specialist mental health services.

Care delivery environments

The environment in which a service is delivered will have a significant impact on the learning opportunities available. Each environment offers unique experiences and can also present specific challenges. This section will highlight some of these points by considering the impact of community and in-patient environments on student learning.

Community placements

The key advantage of many community placements is that they offer you the opportunity to visit people in their own homes. This helps you to gain an insight into how the person's mental health problems are influenced by their environment and social circumstances. It can often provide pieces to the jigsaw puzzle which you would never have known if assessment and contact with the person only happened in an office or a ward environment. Therefore, a more holistic picture is gained of the person by paying attention not only to what they say, but also to your observations of their surroundings and how they interact within their community.

This does, however, have an influence on the dynamics of the relationship you build with the person and how you communicate with them. Most significantly the person is inviting you into their home and, therefore, it is important to respect their rules and routines. In an in-patient setting, the organisation sets the rules and the person who is using the service is expected to adhere to them. In the community, the person is setting the rules and, therefore, you have the opportunity to begin an interaction based on a more equal footing. For example, is there a particular chair that they would rather you sat in? Would they prefer it if you took your shoes off? These simple acts have significant implications for the nature of the relationship you begin to build.

It is also important to remember that the person may not wish to see you that day and, provided that you are not concerned about their safety, they have every right not to allow you into their home. This also reinforces the person's position of choice and emphasises the importance of investing time to engage with the person rather than taking for granted your right to be invited into their personal space.

A further benefit of community placements is the opportunity for you to engage in one-to-one time with the service user without the interruptions or distractions associated with in-patient settings. This can offer you the opportunity to build significant relationships with people and advance your communication skills. You may be encouraged by your mentor to visit someone independently or lead the interaction. This will allow you to take a more active role and move beyond chit-chat to more autonomous and focused interactions. Many students say this opportunity is very beneficial for the development of their confidence as they begin to think of themselves more as a responsible practitioner.

The nature of the one-to-one time you spend with a person can vary widely depending on their current needs and care plan. Students often take advantage of having more time to engage in supporting a person to achieve a specific goal. Some interventions you may be involved in will take place in the community and will be focused on supporting the person to develop independence and confidence or to combat social anxiety. At times, some students find it challenging to see the purpose of their involvement with the person in terms of their learning and feel that they are fulfilling the role of a support worker. It is, therefore, important to be clear about the rationale for the contact you are having with the person so you can ensure you are working within the overall plan of care rather than creating a more socially supportive relationship, which cannot be sustained due to the length of your placement.

The nature of community placements sometimes means that you are not spending as much time in direct contact with service users. This could be because your mentor is completing paperwork, the service user is reluctant for you to visit them or your mentor does not feel it is appropriate for

you to be present. During these periods, some students find it difficult to know how to use this time effectively. In order to combat this, we suggest taking a more self-directed and proactive approach to this placement. Once you have identified the times when you will not be working directly with your mentor, you are then able to approach other members of the team for additional opportunities. Many members of the multidisciplinary team will be very happy to spend time with you or take you with them on visits. You can also use your time to develop your skills in record keeping, becoming familiar with documentation or liaising with other members of the care team. You may also want to organise to visit a service which is linked to the placement area you are in. Whatever you choose, with a little planning you can utilise this time effectively.

In-patient placements

The term 'in-patient area', when used in the context of mental health services, can be taken to mean a setting for mental health care that involves a level of service delivery that is of higher intensity than in a community context. The intensity is heightened in terms of the following aspects:

- Service users are perceived as needing assessment and treatment in a contained setting rather than the service user's home environment.
- The Mental Health Act (1983) may be used at some point during the service user's assessment and treatment.
- Interaction with, and interventions by, a range of mental health professionals is a given.
- The potential for disturbance, annoyance, irritation and aggression from other service users is ever present.
- Opportunities for copycat behaviour and infection by other service users' pathologies are increased.

- Lack of continuity and consistency is an inevitable consequence of the shift systems used in many institutional care settings.
- Activities of daily living such as sleeping, eating, activity and so on may be compromised for most service users in some way.

The student nurse may at first see the above list as intimidating and disadvantageous for their learning opportunities as compared with the more autonomous work setting of the community practitioner. However, you will find that many of your mentors may hold the view that the institutional setting, despite its many disadvantages and discomforts for service users and professional carers, can be a source of similarly intense learning experiences for students. If that idea is applied to the seven areas above, the opportunities for students can be as follows:

- The contained environment is needed to facilitate, primarily, safety and security for the service user. In most instances the reason to assess and treat someone in a hospital environment rather than in their own home means that they are too distressed or disturbed at the time of assessment to be helped in their own home. It is likely, therefore, that the student will see service users being admitted and treated who are often clearly more distressed or disturbed than can be seen in community settings.
- The use of the Mental Health Act (1983) inevitably produces tension between healthcare workers and service users who are being subjected to detention or treatment orders. The ways that experienced and effective professionals strive to maintain therapeutic relationships with service users, despite often being the implementers of the law, can provide rich learning opportunities.
- Institutional healthcare settings, by definition, are sustained by other institutional systems. For example, a typical mental health ward will be serviced by social workers, psychiatrists, occupational therapists, psychologists, phlebotomists, pharmacists, clerks, domestics and so on. The effective mental health nurse must sustain a constructive working relationship with all of these different visitors, in order to provide the best possible service to the client group. As the nurse does this, she provides a role model for the observant student, as well as evidence that the job of a qualified mental health nurse involves skills such as diplomacy, assertiveness and so on, as much as knowledge of medications and Mental Health Act Sections.

◎ Activity

Consider this example:

Student nurse: I've just been sitting with Jim and he says he wants to die . . .

Staff nurse: Oh don't worry. He's always saying that to new staff – especially students.

The very next shift . . .

Student nurse: Hi Jim. How's it going today? You were a bit down yesterday.

Jim: I've really had it. I can't go on like this. You're the only one that seems to be listening to me . . .

The above dialogue illustrates the kind of dilemma that student mental health nurses can easily find themselves in. Do you take Jim's comments at face value, or do you trust the experience of the staff nurse and 'ignore' what he is saying?

Discuss the following with your mentor or other students:

1. What should you, as an individual, do in this situation?
2. How might the 'code of conduct' guide you?

Mental health placement learning areas

Adult community mental health care services

In 1999 the Department of Health published the *National Service Framework for Mental Health* which outlined a new structure for community mental health services. Traditionally community teams worked within a location (often called a catchment area) to provide support to people with a vast variety of problems and at different points in their experiences of distress. In order to promote a recovery approach to delivering community services, a new structure was defined which involved a number of more specialised teams who would focus on specific client groups and provide interventions during defined periods of their distress.

The following section will provide information from students and mentors on these services with a focus on what you should know before commencing the placement, a description of what you might experience and hints and tips on how to make the most of the learning opportunities. Further descriptions of services can be found at the Mind Website (http://www.mind.org.uk).

Placement 1: Crisis intervention and home treatment team: a student experience
Denise Sproat, second-year mental health branch student nurse
The service offers 24-hour crisis intervention and home treatment for people experiencing a severe mental health crisis. People are referred by other services such as their GP and the team are known as the 'gatekeepers' to other services. If the referral meets the criteria initially, the team have to respond within 4 hours and carry out an assessment of the person's mental health. On the whole I found that people presented with thoughts of suicide, or had made an attempt to end their life, and so

were high risk. The service is an alternative to hospital and where a person is taken on by the team they are usually assessed daily over a 72-hour period. Assessments are carried out by two nurses so, as a student, you will be the second person. People are treated at home from anywhere between 2 weeks and 2 months and supported holistically to recovery from their crisis. However, sometimes people can deteriorate and be admitted to hospital.

Melissa Wheeler, second-year mental health branch student nurse
My time as a student nurse with the crisis team was one of the most intense periods of my training within practice. Having the opportunity to work alongside such experienced nurses and multidisciplinary team members on a one-to-one basis was invaluable and made me appreciate the versatility and skills of the team when adapting care to an individual client.

While there I gained a greater understanding of assessments, including mental health examinations, risk assessment and written documentation, and became familiar with a variety of therapeutic approaches and interventions. Time spent with the consultant psychiatrist was extremely rewarding as was attending home visits: both offered opportunities for learning, developed my knowledge base and strengthened my skills of care delivery within changing environments.

I found that many of the crisis team members proved to be supportive role models who were able to facilitate my personal learning and, on reflection, provided me with a greater self-awareness and understanding of others. Although often challenging and hard work, I felt privileged to have been given such a valuable learning opportunity.

Placement 2: Adult community mental health teams (CMHTs)
Rosie Robinson, third-year mental health branch student nurse
In my second year I did two community placements. There are many learning opportunities in a community setting such as working in a team which involves other

Activity

Melissa and Denise identify a number of learning opportunities which they encountered while working with the crisis team. Identify up to three of these learning opportunities which you would prioritise for your placement and consider what prior reading may be helpful in enabling you to achieve these.

Within Melissa and Denise's narratives there may be some roles, definitions or language that you have not heard before. Use the jargon and acronyms buster in Appendices 1 and 2 to identify what these terms mean in a mental health context.

professions such as psychologists, occupational therapists, social workers and psychiatrists. This includes multidisciplinary meetings in which you can participate. I had the opportunity to develop my confidence in administering depot medication. The key learning opportunity for me was that you have the chance to visit people in their own homes and support their carers. I also got much more comfortable with using the Care Programme Approach paperwork, including notes, assessment documentation and care plans along with participating in initial assessments.

I hope you enjoy your community time as much as I did and have a great experience!

 Activity

Rosie describes the benefits of working with the various professionals who work within the CMHT. Before starting your community placement, identify the role of each of these professions and consider how you might benefit from working with them on your placement and what learning outcomes you might achieve.

Placement 3: Early intervention team
Gabriella Maria Burton, second-year mental health branch student nurse
During my second year as a student nurse I got the opportunity to go on placement with an Early Interventions in Psychosis Team. They predominantly work with 15–35-year-olds, suffering with their first untreated psychotic episode. They work to detect early, and intervene to prevent further, damage to the service user's life. This involves intensive work with the service user, families and carers.

Many service users in the service can have a dual diagnosis or no diagnosis at all. This can be many people's first involvement with mental health services and often a very confusing time for them. Due to this, some service users may present angry, scared or confused about the current situation they find themselves in, which is understandable, so you need to educate, support and empathise with them. Although saying this, many service users have been with the team for some time and have built a therapeutic relationship with their care coordinator and there will be various people that you can work closely with and build your own therapeutic relationship with.

There are many learning opportunities as there are so many different professionals in the team such as family therapists and cognitive behavioural therapists. Opportunities I came across incorporated initial assessments, depots, social groups, care plan reviews, social circumstance reports and many more interventions.

 Reflection point

Gabriella describes how a person might feel who is experiencing psychosis for the first time and the importance of empathising with their experience.

1. How might you feel if you were in the service user's position?
2. How might this influence how you work with the person?

Placement 4: Assertive outreach team
Amy Ramful, third-year mental health branch student nurse

During my second year of training I had a placement with the Assertive Outreach Community Team. Assertive Outreach work with service users with severe and enduring mental illness who have difficulties engaging with services. Some service users may also have a forensic background or dual diagnosis. The team tends to have smaller case loads compared to a CMHT, which allows for more intensive treatment which helps with engagement issues.

As a student, don't be surprised if some service users aren't keen on having you involved in their care. This is the nature of the client group. When I first started the placement my mentor told me to expect a lot of unanswered doors and running around trying to get hold of people. However, don't let this put you off because, of the work the team does with clients, many have built very good therapeutic relationships with the team, and there will be plenty of opportunities for you to work closely with some of them, and you may even have the chance to have your own mini caseload.

Other learning opportunities I came across included depot administration, Care Programme Approach reviews, risk assessments, Mental Health Act assessments, care planning and doing individual work with service users.

◖◗ Reflection point

Amy describes the challenges of working with people who are reluctant to have students involved in their care.

1. Why do you think this might be the case?
2. Think about how you would make the most of your time on placement during periods when you are not having contact with service users.
3. What type of approach might help people feel comfortable with having you involved in their care?

Adult 24-hour care services

A key aim of the *National Service Framework for Mental Health* (Department of Health 1999) was to design services which provide mental health care in the least restrictive environment. Over the past 30 years the number of hospital beds has significantly decreased and every effort is made to support people who are in distress to remain in their own homes. This model of mental health care aims to reduce the disruption a period of crisis may have to a person's life and limit the effects of continuous admission to hospital. People who have previously experienced this type of care are often referred to as 'revolving door patients'. This label inevitably has negative connotations for the person's potential for recovery.

There are, however, times when hospital admission is thought to be unavoidable. This may be due to the person's safety towards themselves or others or due to requiring assessment and treatment under Section 2 or 3 of the Mental Health Act. Alternatively, a person may have recovered from their period of crisis but require additional support to enable them to regain the skills, roles and relationships required for them to move on from mental health services. In these circumstances the following 24-hour care services are available.

Placement 5: Crisis admission, treatment and therapy ward (acute ward)
Sharon Taylor, third-year mental health branch student nurse

My placement on an acute in-patient ward proved to be the most challenging, stimulating and rewarding experience in my student career. Generally speaking, people are admitted to the ward at their most distressed and vulnerable, and for a short period of time. This meant the ward was often busy and intense with a high patient turnover. I learnt a lot about the power of human kindness in bringing comfort to people; listening with compassionate understanding to people's lived experience of illness, treatment and recovery; and what it means to be a patient on an acute ward. This helped me to develop a more responsive approach to individual patient care.

I liked and benefited from the pace and variety of experiences acute nursing offers; one minute I could be doing a depot, the next minute an MDT, then reading patients their rights under the Mental Health Act. I enjoyed being part of the team; working with other health professionals was inspiring and taught me what it means to work collaboratively, particularly approaching problem solving and risk management as a shared experience.

 Activity

> Sharon tells us that she was involved in 'reading patients their rights under the Mental Health Act'. Use the links in Chapter 3 and discussion with your mentor to find out what she means by this and what it would entail.

Placement 6: Psychiatric intensive care unit
Tanya Ames, third-year mental health branch student nurse
Often students are apprehensive about a placement on a psychiatric intensive care unit (PICU). This is often due to having a limited knowledge, being misinformed and having negative preconceived ideas. After feeling particularly fearful and nervous about this placement, I reluctantly agreed and, in hindsight, it has been an invaluable placement experience.

The PICU where I was placed provides 24-hour care in a low-stimulus environment for 20 males aged 18–65, accommodated on two sides and contained within a secure, locked unit: side A (8 intensive care beds) and side B (12 forensic rehabilitation beds). Side A manages patients who need initial assessment, high levels of nursing intervention and exhibit challenging behaviour. Side B is a low-security unit offering ongoing assessments and support for patients needing longer term treatment or preparation for resettlement.

Care and treatment are provided for those who cannot be managed on acute wards or other settings such as prisons. The service users are assessed as presenting a high risk to themselves or others and are at risk of absconding. The majority of patients have a primary diagnosis of a psychosis, many have a secondary diagnosis such as substance misuse and many have a forensic history. Most patients are detained on Section 3 of the Mental Health Act. As there are a limited number of beds, the staff:patient ratio is very high, as are levels of observation. 'Incidents' are infrequent, and any which do occur are quickly and effectively contained.

There are plenty of opportunities to meet practice outcomes/competencies such as liaising with other agencies, forming and maintaining therapeutic relationships with patients and their families, accurately recording documentation, undertaking initial and ongoing assessments, monitoring patients on high-observation levels, dispensing oral medication and administering depot injections, participating in ward rounds and multidisciplinary team meetings. Additional learning opportunities include insight visits to local prisons, acute wards and observing electroconvulsive treatment.

Although I had initially viewed my impending placement with trepidation, it soon became apparent that my fears were unjustified. The nursing team was very welcoming and supportive, understood my apprehension and soon put my mind at rest. My advice would be to start this placement with an open mind and take advantage of all the learning opportunities available to you.

⟨⟩ Reflection point

Tanya describes feeling worried about working with this client group due to some preconceived ideas. She identifies how she worked with the team to overcome and challenge these perceptions in order to gain a valuable learning experience.

1. Do you have similar concerns or worries about working with a specific client group?
2. What support is available to you to explore these worries?
3. How might you consider ways of managing your worries to enable you to make the most of your learning experience?

Placement 7: Residential rehabilitation and recovery services

Emily Trivett, third-year mental health branch student nurse

During my first year I started my placement in a rehabilitation community unit. The placement itself was a house set in the community that provided accommodation for adults with mental health problems. The setting allowed the people to be surrounded
by a nursing team, complete with occupational therapists, healthcare assistants and a cook. People come to learn new skills and master skills they have lost, such as learning to cook, clean and do their own washing – something we take for granted.

I was able to get fully involved with the nursing staff and actually help the patients to learn valuable skills during their stay. The patients stay normally for an assessment process of 8 weeks and this is reviewed to see how they have managed and whether they can move on to independent living. This is the aim for all the residents who reside at the house. Some come for 2 weeks at a time and come for the staying-well

programme (SWP) to keep them well and to prevent relapse.

The service user develops a programme of what activities they are expected to do for the week, a combination of cooking their own meals, going on walks, budgeting when buying ingredients and using public transport. Also they are required to attend in-house meetings and do activities within the house, such as tidying their rooms, doing their washing and cleaning up after they have cooked meals.

I was able to experience what it is like working closely with people, encouraging them to make their own meals and motivating them to try new things. I gave them ideas for what they could cook and assessed their ability to cook on their own. I also took part in art and crafts, and ran my own groups with some of the staff. I also accompanied the service users on walks to parks and to shops to buy cooking ingredients.

The placement allowed me to be able to complete paperwork and do certain tasks on my own, once I had seen them done by someone else, such as completing risk assessments, admission forms, etc. I thoroughly enjoyed this placement as it enabled me to feel fully involved with both the team of staff and the service users. It was also a chance for me to begin to understand how mental health nurses work and to be involved with different professionals such as doctors and occupational therapists.

⟨⟩ Reflection point

Emily describes being involved in supporting people to develop skills which will enable them to live independently. This type of work is often known as promoting social inclusion.

1. What do you understand by this term?
2. What might it entail?
3. How might you be involved in promoting social inclusion as a student mental health nurse?

Older adult mental health care services

Older adult mental healthcare services provide assessment and treatment to people over the age of 65. People who access the service may have the types of mental health issues you would see in adult care settings such as low mood, anxiety, psychosis or poor coping strategies. These are often referred to in this practice area as functional mental health problems. Some people will have developed these issues in the later years of their life, however some may have been involved with mental health services for many years. Alternatively, people may require support from mental health services due to issues resulting from deterioration in the function of the brain such as memory problems, dementia and Alzheimer's disease. These are often termed organic mental health problems.

Placement 8: 24-hour care assessment units
Charlotte Kawalek, third-year mental health branch student nurse

As a first-year student, with some prior experience in the mental health field, I felt going into an elderly in-patient admission ward was a brilliant opportunity for me to be able to gain a basic grounding into a range of mental health problems and what effect they had on the individual and the carers and, indeed, how the nursing staff and others within the multidisciplinary team interacted with the client, as part of their treatment.

When most people hear 'elderly', they have visions of people who are physically unwell and who require a lot of help with their personal care. While this can be true, the reality is that they too are people, who have complex mental health needs which can be accompanied by these physical ailments, but these are certainly not the beginning and end of in-patient care for the elderly. The wards do tend to be busy places but they are a great place to gain the basic principles of patient care which are fundamental to nursing.

The key learning opportunities I experienced were, first, completing assessment documentation (from taking people's life history and physical health checks to completing risk screens and care plans). I found these provide a great basis for the whole of the nursing course, and the earlier you get involved in completing them, the more comfortable you are in asking people questions, and developing your own style for completing the documentation. I found observing lots of nurses complete this process very helpful, as it allows you to reflect upon the parts you thought worked well/did not work well so you can develop in your own practice as your confidence and experience grow.

I also developed an understanding of the Mental Health Act. This is a really good placement to look into the Mental Health Act and all of the different Sections, so take all opportunities to see any assessments and regarding of Sections as they provide an invaluable experience.

There are lots of opportunities for taking physical observations in this placement area. These opportunities do not come about as often as I certainly expected, so my advice would be to grasp the opportunity to practise taking people's baseline observations whenever possible, as it is all important to nursing care. I also found looking at medications and their side effects useful in relation to physical health, such as hypertension, which is certainly common in the elderly but it can also be a side effect of medication so it is important to ask about these.

In relation to personal care, the issues of maintaining privacy and dignity of the clients was really important and also gaining consent for permission to be involved in people's care. This all required me to develop my communication skills both with the people who were using the service and the multidisciplinary team.

Placement 9: Older adult community mental health services
Charlotte Kawalek, third-year mental health branch student nurse

While this area differs from the ward-based placements, it too has many elements in common, and personally was a fantastic placement, allowing me to develop my skills as a practitioner and to increase my confidence in assessments leading to me completing a number of these with little assistance and doing home visits alone.

It is a great place to be able to really get stuck in and apply all that is taught in university and how this can be applied in the context of people's own homes. It can be challenging, but is also a very stimulating area to work.

The placement offers many opportunities. First, to see how people cope in their own home and to offer support to enable them to continue doing this. The development of working relationships is vital as there are normally a number of professionals involved and it is all good management skills. The assessment process and assessing risk is slightly different and it's good to ask mentors to explain this to you, as it is their role if they are care coordinator. The placement also offered a range of experiences seeing individuals with functional and organic illness, and involved close working with carers, which enabled development of communication skills.

Placement 10: Older adult day hospital
Charlotte Kawalek, third-year mental health branch student nurse

This is often thought of as 'day care' and can be viewed in a negative light; where people view their main role as providing a few activities, tea and biscuits. However, my experience of working at a day hospital was very different to this assumption.

I found that it was a professionally challenging placement, if you apply what you have learnt over the course of your training to the placement area. I found I was able to complete assessments, work effectively within the multidisciplinary team and apply evidence-based research into practice, which is a fundamental component of nursing today. It was also a brilliant way of again developing interpersonal skills and learning to work as an effective member of the multidisciplinary team, working alongside community psychiatric nurses, the wards and occupational therapists within the team. It also allowed me to attend many review meetings where families were involved and to be able to see how the different services within mental health services all complemented each other and how they work together to aim to provide holistic care.

I learnt that the role of the day hospital is to provide different activities dependent on the client group. On days where people with organic problems attended, the days tended to focus on providing meaningful occupation, including reminiscent activities, exercises and promoting the maintenance of independent living skills; along with assessing clients for day care, or alternative services as a form of respite for carers. On the days where people with functional problems attended, we tended to focus on promoting independent living skills and rehabilitation on a small scale for people, as an interim often between hospital and home.

The day hospital also provided occupation in meaningful activities, but these tended to be focused on art activities and management of different mental illnesses as a form of education for the clients. Furthermore, a memory clinic also ran at the day hospital, which provided assessment of individuals referred to the service by their GP. In addition, a memory support group ran where individuals could attend after being newly diagnosed with a memory problem in order to provide them with education about the illness and planning for the future.

Activity

Charlotte describes three different placement settings which involve working with older adults. From her descriptions and discussion with your mentor, try to identify what factors would be considered when assessing which service would be most beneficial to the older adult. You may wish to consider both social and healthcare needs.

Forensic services

Placement 11: Secure 24-hour care settings

Lucy Mangnall, third-year mental health branch student nurse

During my third year I was given the opportunity to have a placement at a high-security forensic special hospital as part of my complex needs placement.

I found the learning opportunities available at this placement were vast and included the chance to spend one-on-one time with psychiatrists and gain a more in-depth understanding of their role. I had opportunities to learn basic pharmacology and relate it to psychotropic medication. I also contributed highly to the care of my mentor's caseload. Along with taking part and taking the lead in ward rounds, security liaison meetings and Care Programme Approach reviews, I also developed my knowledge of the relevant sections of the Mental Health Act and how this was implemented in this area.

A key area in this setting is around risk management and risk reduction and I was able to gain experiences in working with individual patients who had severely challenging behaviours. This may involve escorting a patient outside of the secure area and the difficulties that this imposes, managing a patient who has been assessed as requiring high levels of observation and also observing how the nurse manages a patient in seclusion.

 Activity

Lucy describes observing how the nurse manages a patient in seclusion.

1. What is your understanding of this term?
2. What does the seclusion policy state in your healthcare trust?
3. When do you think this would be a justified intervention?
4. What are your perceptions of seclusion as an intervention?
5. What do your student colleagues think about seclusion as an intervention?

Complex care settings

Clinical areas of this nature provide interventions and approaches which are developed to meet the needs of a specific client group or mental health difficulty. They often involve nurses and healthcare professionals who have undertaken further education in approaches which are adopted in these areas. Many work in conjunction with other mental health services to give specialist input or provide components of the person's care. The range of these types of services is vast and continuously growing in both the statutory and private sector. Below are some of the most common types of complex care settings which are most likely to be available in your area.

Placement 12: Substance misuse services

Tony Moore, third-year mental health branch student nurse

I spent my specialist placement with the substance misuse service, primarily on a 13-bed in-patient drug and alcohol detox ward, which specialises in drug detoxification and stabilisation and alcohol detoxification. I have always had an interest in substance misuse and people with substance misuse problems. Unlike other placements I undertook, mental health issues, if present, are secondary to substance misuse issues but are still monitored and addressed when necessary. I found the client group extremely interesting and generally they were more than happy to discuss their life and the circumstances that led them to misuse drugs and alcohol. As a student mental health nurse, I was anticipating stories of self-medication for mental health issues, tragic life events and deprived upbringing. Although this is the case with some of the patients, I found that the majority of people took drugs and drank because they enjoyed it but it had become problematic with extensive use.

The ward provides an excellent opportunity to understand the types of illicit drugs used and the process of addiction, detoxification and the medication used, stabilisation on opiate substitutes and blockers. As the ward has only 13 beds and the patients are admitted for between 7 and 21 days, there is ample opportunity to form therapeutic relationships, and by the end of the placement you should be able to perform preadmission assessments and devise individual treatment plans for patients. One of the most difficult aspects of the placement, in my opinion, is trying to convince a patient, who wishes to self-discharge before completing treatment, to stay on the ward. This can be very challenging if the patient, is craving drugs or alcohol as they will be very fixated on this and it can be extremely difficult to talk them around. A real positive aspect is seeing both the physical and mental improvement in people as the treatment, progresses and this can be very rewarding. Although the field of substance misuse may not be 'proper' mental health, it is an interesting and progressive service and makes an excellent placement.

Placement 13: Child and adolescent services
Tim Westwood, third-year mental health branch student nurse

I found child and adolescent mental health services (CAMHS) a strange place when I started my placement as it was so different to adult placements I had been on. I was amazed at the absence of clients with diagnoses. Where were the schizophrenics, clinically depressed and the personality disorders? The truth was that children usually don't have a diagnosis as there is no benefit in giving children adult labels. What you are left with is the sad children, the angry children and the 'not doing as well as they should be' children.

The absence of a diagnosis means that treatment is non-medication based and the most surprising thing of all is that the first treatment offered is not for the child at all but for their parents. Parents are offered training on how best to support their child. Talking treatments then focus on the family dynamics and identifying any traumatic events that have occurred in the child's life. Treatment is a long-term commitment for the family and CAMHS. The symptoms of childhood mental distress I observed included poor concentration levels at school, anger towards parents and siblings, hyperactivity and nightmares.

What you get with a CAMHS placement is a chance to work with individuals at the early stages of mental distress. You will be working with the unformed mind and success at this stage could prevent the child enduring mental illness in the future. It is a challenging placement as dealing with childhood distress is difficult. You will hear stories that will

---

 Activity

Tony describes his placement working with a substance misuse team, however we have also heard other students talk about working with people with a 'dual diagnosis'. This often refers to people who have a mental health problem and a substance misuse problem. The link between the two is contentious and there is a high level of debate surrounding this issue.

1. How do you think substance misuse can impact on mental health?
2. What is your impression of what the media say about how substances can affect mental health?
3. Discuss this with your mentor and identify how the media might influence your perception towards people with a dual diagnosis and the way you would work with them.

break your heart but, saying that, I can't recommend it enough and it is an experience not to be missed.

⟨⟩ Reflection point

Tim describes finding working with children personally challenging as a result of working with children in distress. It is evident, however, that he found this experience a valuable learning opportunity.

In order to prepare for a placement working with children, what might you need to consider in terms of your own support needs?

Placement 14: Mental health liaison teams

Ben Thompson, first-year mental health branch student nurse, and Keith Waters, mental health liaison team leader

A placement with the mental health liaison team offers a wide range of learning opportunities, with exposure to a full spectrum of mental health presentations, often occurring in crisis, many of which will be coming into contact with services for the first time. It provides an excellent chance to develop and consolidate assessment and diagnosis skills, and regular exposure to risk management and recommending treatment options. The team works largely in isolation although there is some multidisciplinary working with other mental health services. However, there is regular interaction with colleagues operating within the general hospital setting including exposure to areas of general nursing you would not normally see, including the emergency department, medical wards and intensive care units.

The placement can be emotionally demanding as the student is often working with clients who are experiencing extreme emotional distress. In many ways it is a privilege to be present and influential at what is a

pivotal life event for many clients and it can be rewarding when clients express gratitude for the assistance and support the team provides. The work of the team is also well received and much respected by medical staff in the hospital who may have minimal mental health training and can find managing mental health clients an anxious and difficult experience.

The workload on the team is variable and unpredictable which means there are quiet times. Take this opportunity to pick up on any questions you may have, or to do some background reading. The flip side of this is that at busy times you may not always get away on time.

⟨⟩ Reflection point

Ben describes how this placement offered him the opportunity to work with colleagues from the adult field of nursing in settings such as the emergency department. Before commencing your placement, reflect with your student colleagues on the following points:

1. If you have mental health problems or are extremely emotionally distressed, how might you feel in the emergency room environment?

2. How might this influence the way you might act or respond to healthcare professionals?

3. What approaches might be helpful when working with a person with mental health problems in this environment? You might want to consider:

   a. your initial manner when you meet the person for the first time
   b. the environment you speak with them in
   c. the information you give them about yourself and the purpose of you talking with them.

Placement 15: Motherhood and mental health

Charlotte Bridges, third-year mental health branch student nurse

The mother and baby ward is an acute mental health ward that cares for mothers that have become mentally unwell or relapsed due to pregnancy or birth. On the ward that I was on, the mother and baby come to the ward together – the mother is not admitted without the baby. The criteria are that the baby must be under 7 months old and mothers are admitted during pregnancy. The ward and the mother and baby community team work very closely together to ensure that all staff are informed of potential admissions or supported discharges. The aim of the service is to provide a safe environment for the mother and baby that aids the recovery of the mother, promotes bonding between mother and baby and offers support and advice about care of the baby. This is done by medication, therapies/interventions, support and education.

The placement has really opened my eyes to working with positive risk. The mothers need to keep contact with their babies to aid with the bonding process, however, when a mother is mentally unwell, this can pose many risks to the baby. This is also applicable when breastfeeding; some medications advise that mothers don't breastfeed therefore you need to look at whether they really need that medication or whether they can change to a different one and consider the different debates that arise from this type of dilemma.

Advice for students from Polly Murray, a staff nurse working in a mother and baby in-patient unit

- Look at the mother's care plans and talk to staff about how much support is needed with baby care. Some women may require lots of support to meet their baby's needs; others may request lots of help but may actually be more capable then they think they are. In the latter instances, you may feel that you are helping by 'taking over' baby care, however it is not necessarily in the mother or baby's best interests. Intervening can reduce the mother's confidence, prevent maternal bonds from forming and, if this is maintained, there is even a danger that the baby may start to bond with you. Instead, offer to stay with the mother, talk her through the task in hand and reinforce how capable she is.
- Try to have a basic understanding of maternity issues and baby care prior to starting the placement, or get someone to explain issues (such as feeding, weaning, winding and changing nappies) to you at

 Activity

Charlotte mentions that medication is used to help mothers recover from the mental health problems they are experiencing. Some medications are not used if the woman is pregnant or breastfeeding, due to the potential harm they could cause the baby.

Use the *British National Formulary* (BNF) 2011 and discussion with your mentor to identify these medications and what alternative medications or interventions are used.

There are some mental health problems which are only experienced by women who are pregnant or have had a baby, such as postnatal depression and puerperal psychosis.

Use the *International Classification of Mental and Behavioural Disorder* (ICD) 10 and discussion with your mentor to identify what these mental health problems are and how a person who is experiencing one of these problems may act and feel.

the start of the placement. Maybe look back at your documentation from your maternity placements.

- The majority of women who use the unit do not pose ongoing/significant risks to their children, however occasionally referrals will be made to social services regarding safeguarding issues. This is a great opportunity for students to learn how to assess risk, make referrals to children's services, the role of children's services and how social and mental health services support families to reduce such risks.
- Attend allocations meetings where the community team discusses new referrals to the service. This will give you a good understanding of the referral criteria and the variety of mental health problems which the service caters for.
- Organise to go on home visits with specialist perinatal community psychiatric nurses. This will develop your understanding of assessments, the different presentations of women treated at home and in hospital and how risk is managed in the community.

◑ Reflection point

Polly advises students to have a basic understanding of maternity issues and baby care before starting the placement.

Consider how you might gain this understanding and make an action plan on how you will achieve this.

Placement 16: Psychotherapy
Sarah Moore, third-year mental health branch student nurse
As a third-year student and having an interest in cognitive behavioural therapy for some years, I felt gaining a placement with a psychological

therapies service was an invaluable opportunity for me to be able to gain experience in how different therapies work and what sort of mental health problems they are particularly useful for. The service employed counsellors, psychodynamic therapists, low-intensity cognitive behavioural therapists and high-intensity cognitive behavioural therapists.

Some people may think therapies are about a client talking and the therapist listening. Listening is a key skill in any therapy but by no means is this the be all and end all. With any therapy it is about gathering information about the client and details of what the problem is, sometimes supporting the client to find where the problem lies. However, all therapies are underlined with different theories and these alter the techniques used by different therapists.

My main aim when on placement was to find out more about cognitive behavioural therapy, the theories that underline it, how it is used and what mental health problems it works best with. During my time I had the opportunity to discover these. Other learning opportunities included completing assessment documentation (from taking people's life histories, important events, mental and physical questions, risk screening and treatment plans). The more of this you get involved with the more comfortable you become with carrying it out. This would be called gradual exposure and is actually a cognitive behavioural technique used in anxiety-related problems. Different practitioners have different methods of completing assessments and observing many has helped develop the way I prefer to carry them out.

Being involved in providing therapy is definitely a great opportunity to develop communication skills such as verbal, listening, body language and even knowing when to divert away from a particular subject when it is too much for the client.

I was able to understand how different therapies worked and why different therapies worked better with some mental health problems than others. I had a great experience and I plan on doing my cognitive behavioural training in the near future.

Activity

Sarah describes the use of a number of therapies in the area that she was placed and how it is useful to have a basic understanding of these and the models that underpin them.

1. Identify one of these therapies and use this book to find out more about it and how it is used (Ch. 3 and Sect. 2 might be particularly useful).
2. Look up one of the recommended reading texts, for the therapy you have chosen, to expand your knowledge further.

Placements 17: Voluntary sector
Mark Lambert, Team Leader,
Framework Housing Association

Placements in the voluntary sector are very different to placements within a NHS setting, because a person's mental health and how that is managed is not the primary focus of the support provided. The support provided within the voluntary sector focuses on the practical aspects of daily living/issues while taking into account how a person's mental health can impact on their ability to manage these issues. Therefore, within these placement settings, you get to see the whole person as an individual and not just the person and their illness.

Voluntary services are based in a community setting and are reliant upon developing good lines of communication with statutory services which are responsible for supporting people with their mental health. The voluntary services are typically hostels which provide support housing solutions or floating support services which support people in their own homes. Services such as these are typically funded from central government funds that are prioritised to area of need as defined by individual local authorities. (This is not inclusive of all voluntary sector organisations but is true for those that are funded to provide support around housing/independent living.)

The support in services funded in this manner focuses on housing needs, money management – budgeting, debt, maximising income, getting into work – and social inclusion.

As the voluntary sector is based within a community setting you meet people who are at differing stages of their recovery and are therefore linked in to differing statutory services which you would liaise with (i.e. acute wards, CMHTs, day centres, out-patient clinics).

You also have the opportunity to support people to contact benefit agencies, housing departments and agencies connected to debt (be that specialist support agencies, a person's creditors, debt collectors, etc.). This will enable you to gain a good insight into the aspects of daily living that impact upon a person's mental health and how a person's mental health impacts on their ability to manage situations and their day-to-day life.

Currently services in the voluntary sector are privileged to be able to spend a greater amount of time with individuals than workers within community mental health teams, therefore grasp this opportunity.

 Activity

Mark recognises that the learning opportunities you may encounter in the voluntary sector may be different to those in the NHS. Explore with your personal tutor the following:

1. What alternative opportunities might this offer you as a student on placement?
2. How will you ensure you achieve your learning outcomes in an area which is less focused on medical interventions and where nurses are not the predominant profession?

Top tips

The following top tips are from student mental health nurses and aim to help you make the most out of your mental health placement.

Communication skills

- Listen more than you talk – every service user's story will be different.
- Take the time to sit and talk with the service users. Yes, there's always paperwork that needs doing but find time to get back to basics. Service users will remember those who sat and listened to them.

Placement support

- Use the supervision offered to discuss any issues that arise during the placement – it can be distressing to hear service users talk about their experiences.
- Seek support from your mentor or personal tutor if you experience difficult or challenging situations that have the potential to affect you in a negative way.

Attitude

- The main thing which is helpful is respecting the service user as an individual and seeing past the diagnosis.
- Don't make assumptions or have preconceived ideas based upon what you have heard or been told. Remain open minded and make your own judgements based upon your own personal experiences of the placement.
- Empathise, don't judge. Try and understand how they are feeling and put yourself in their situation. Showing someone you care means so much.

Approach

- A good way of developing effective therapeutic relationships is through working on documenting the person's life history. This provides insight into the

person and allows care to be more holistic.
- Speaking to carers/family members is also a key role of the nurse. Also it allows you a deeper insight into the service and, thus, you are able to engage them in holistic care as you have a greater understanding of them as a person.

Enhancing learning opportunities

- Remember that, as with every placement, you will get out of it what you put into it. See each day and every opportunity as a new learning experience. You only have the chance to be a student nurse once!
- Know what you want from this placement – the opportunities are there for the taking.
- Learn from the good practice of existing staff.
- Opt for a variety of shifts to become familiar with the different dynamics of working environments. Also at weekends there will be more time for discussion and learning support.
- Use reflective practice within portfolio work to reflect on and establish your new learning – you'll be surprised at how many aspects of learning you cover in a day.
- Answer the office telephone. This gives you the opportunity to engage with a range of multiagencies. Following up on jobs created through this process will create opportunities for further learning.
- Don't be afraid to take a lead and ask your mentor and the rest of the team if there are any suitable service users for you to work with as a named nurse.
- Volunteer to do the notes. The nurse will appreciate the help with the paperwork and you will learn how to document and think about what this means for your accountability. Read previous entries to see how others have written and documented their contacts.
- If you feel confident, ask to do more. It may seem daunting, but things such as

speaking up in the multidisciplinary meetings and actually taking the lead in initial assessments will build your confidence and give you the experiences you need.

- In the community, the car journeys are a great time to ask questions about your mentor's experiences as a nurse and current issues in mental health. Mentors prefer students who are inquisitive and want to learn.
- Be prepared to challenge and educate people's current views – this could be a service user, family member or anyone involved in the service user's care.
- Try to do some background reading of the assessment approaches, theories and models that underpin different therapies.
- Be prepared for quiet times – have a book to hand and keep a list of questions for reference that you may not have had a chance to ask at the time.
- Revise your knowledge of sections of the Mental Health Act and the Mental Capacity Act and look at the duty of care under common law and broader ethical issues.
- Go on visits with as many different members of the team as possible. As everyone works differently, you will get to witness lots of different styles and see how people have to adapt to different clients.

Working effectively with your mentor
The following questions aim to help you develop a shared understanding with your mentor of the mentorship process and how it will work in your individual circumstances. These questions should be discussed within the first week of placement and completed as a record of your agreement which you can revisit and revise throughout.

- What are our expectations of each other?
- What are our expectations of the mentoring process?
- How often will we plan to meet both formally and informally?

- How will we communicate in between meetings?
- What time will be available for learning individually in the workplace?
- How will feedback be given on aspects of my practice?
- How will we organise additional support following a challenging situation?
- Are there any other areas that we feel are important to identify to support learning in this placement area?

Action planning

As you move through your programme you will become increasingly aware of your developing learning needs. It is important to define these and communicate them to your mentor. It is also an effective skill for the future as it will encourage you to be a more self-directive learner and less reliant on your mentor to identify learning opportunities. Here are some suggestions of things you may want to think about:

Professional development
- What are the priorities for learning that I have already identified from previous placements?
- Which competencies am I focused upon achieving?
- What immediate learning opportunities are there in this practice area that will enable me to meet these competencies?
- What additional learning opportunities will I need to seek elsewhere to enable me to meet these competencies?
- What support will I need from the team to settle into the practice area and achieve my competencies?
- What evidence will demonstrate I have achieved these competencies?

Clinical development
- How will I engage with current service users in the practice area?

Table 4.1 Summary of learning needs and action plan

What is my specific learning goal?	What resources or support do I need to meet this goal?	How will I know when I have met this goal?	When will I review progress with my mentor?
1.			
2.			
3.			

- How will I develop my independence and confidence in this practice area?
- How will I enhance my confidence in clinical skills?
- What are the specific clinical skills that I am concerned about?
- How will I enhance my skills and confidence in leadership and case management?

Personal development
- What are my career aspirations and how will I work towards these?
- What are the practice development opportunities I would like to be involved in?
- How will I develop professional networks relevant to my role?
- How will my progress in this area contribute to my portfolio?

For each of the learning needs you identify you should consider the questions given in Table 4.1 and summarise your answers to discuss with your mentor.

References

Darzi, A., 2008. High quality care for all. NHS next stage review final report, summary. Department of Health, London.

Department of Health, 1999. National service framework for mental health: modern standards and service models. HMSO, London.

Longley, M., Shaw, C., Dolan, G., 2007. Nursing: towards 2015. Alternative scenarios for healthcare, nursing and nurse education in the UK in 2015. Welsh Institute for Health and Social Care, Pontypridd.

Nursing and Midwifery Council, 2010. Standards for pre-registration education. NMC, London.

Further reading

Biernacki, C., 2007. Dementia: metamorphosis in care. John Wiley & Sons, West Sussex.

Dogra, N., Leighton, S. (Eds.), 2009. Nursing in child and adolescent mental health. Blackwell,Oxford.

Dogra, N., Parkin, A., Gale, F., Frake, C. (Eds.), 2008. A multi-disciplinary handbook of child and adolescent mental health for front-line professionals, 2nd ed. Jessica Kingsley, London.

Kitwood, T., 1997. Dementia reconsidered: the person comes first (rethinking aging). Open University Press, Buckingham.

Levett-Jones, T., Bourgeois, S., 2009. The clinical placement: a nursing survival guide, 2nd ed. Elsevier, London.

McDougall, T. (Ed.), 2006. Child and adolescent mental health nursing. Blackwell, Oxford.

McGarry, J., Clissett, P., Porrock, D., (In press). Pocket placement guide for care of the older person. Elsevier, London.

Royal Pharmaceutical Society, 2010. British National Formulary 61. Pharmaceutical Press, London. Online. Available at: http://bnf.org/bnf/bnf/current (accessed June 2011).

Sharples, K., 2009. Learning to learn in practice. Learning Matters, Exeter.

World Health Organisation, 2007. International classification of mental and behavioural disorder (ICD) 10. WHO, Geneva. Online. Available at:http://apps. who.int/classifications/apps/icd/ icd10online (accessed June 2011).

5 The practicalities of mental health placements

CHAPTER AIMS

• To help you to prepare for placements in a mental health setting

Introduction

This chapter aims to provide possible answers or solutions to common questions students have about the practicalities of mental health placements. It will help you to prepare for your placement in a mental health setting and prompt you to identify the information you will need to gather from the specific area you are going to.

You should also refer to the list of acronyms in Appendix 1 and the jargon buster in Appendix 2 for a glossary of terms used in this area of practice in order to help you to feel more prepared and confident when embarking on a new placement.

Practical issues for students going to new placements

Dress code

Contact the placement prior to arriving for your first day. Do not assume that the care staff don't wear uniform because they are based in the community *or* do wear uniform because they are based in a hospital. There are exceptions to both these generalisations, and culture and philosophy in mental healthcare settings often change. For example, some recent changes back into uniform have been driven by the need to control the spread of infection more effectively, rather than as an attempt to clearly demarcate professional carers from service users. (The use of alcohol hand gels, implemented for exactly the same reason, has brought with it difficult consequences such as ingestion by mental health service users (Archer 2007, Bairy 2006, Batty et al 2011).)

Another issue to consider is the need to present a professional image. Exactly what this means can only be gleaned by looking at what your colleagues are wearing. Some areas will be happy for you to wear jeans, whereas others will consider this inappropriate. Your work area is not the place to be making fashion statements. Your job is to be as approachable as professionally possible. Your clothing should not be a barrier to your achievement of this. Wear clothing which is comfortable but also appropriately formal or informal.

The Nursing and Midwifery Council (NMC) *Guidance on Professional Conduct for Nursing and Midwifery Students* states that students need to 'follow the dress code or uniform policy of your university and clinical placement provider' (NMC 2009). The most useful way to interpret this guidance is, as mentioned above, to emulate the dress standards of your professional colleagues. Usually any misinterpretation on your part will be quickly pointed out by a colleague on the placement.

This guidance also applies to culturally sensitive issues in your work with service users. Be aware that, for example, tattoos, piercings and florid artificial hair colourings may serve to distance the very people that you are trying to engage with. Again, be welcoming of advice from your mentors about this if it seems to be an issue.

Some things to do before, and during, your placement

- Telephone for an appointment to visit the placement and, if possible, meet your new mentor (this can help to alleviate or validate your preplacement anxiety).
- Decide to make up your own mind about the placement based on your own real experience – not what you hear from others.
- Ensure you know what your shifts are, and be on time.
- Ensure you have the appropriate competency paperwork with you and that you have thought about what you would like to achieve during the placement – this can always be altered if you change your mind.
- Read journal articles and search the Internet for background information about the type of clinical environment you are about to experience.
- If you are happy with your placement experience, make sure that you tell your mentor.
- If you are unhappy with it, tell your mentor. Do not wait until the end of the

placement or, worse still, have left it. If this is in any way difficult for you, get support.
- The effectiveness of your mentor will fundamentally affect the experience you have in your placement. Decide to invest in the relationship you have with them, even though it is relatively transient.
- Attempt to be empathic towards your mentor. Most have increasingly difficult demands on them in the current economic climate. To be an effective mentor takes commitment, initiative, flexibility and energy.

Making the most of time with your mentor

This does not mean being with your mentor all the time you are on duty. Some of your richest learning may come from the time that you are not with your mentor. Set the situation up to help both of you. Be an asset to your mentor rather than a part of their caseload. Be proactive as well as reactive. Work to create opportunities for yourself to enhance your learning in each placement. If the placement is not your ideal, then discuss this with your mentor. Try to make the best of each experience you have. Be memorable for the right reasons.

What to expect from your mentor
- A positive role model, in terms of behaviour, attitude and professionalism.
- Empathy with what it is to be a student.
- Empathy with what it is to be you.
- To be a resource and a sign-poster to resources.
- Honesty.
- Congruence.
- Welcoming – even though you will undoubtedly represent extra work for them.

- Up to date in terms of evidence-based practice.
- Open to innovative suggestions from you, regarding care practices.

 Activity

1. In small groups, list the characteristics of an *effective* mentor.
2. Use the following link to look up the standards for supporting learning and assessment in practice which were published by the NMC in 2010:
   - http://www.nmc-uk.org/ Publications/Standards (accessed June 2011)
3. How do these standards compare to your list of characteristics?

Lone-working policies

Community-based placements will have agreed and accessible policies to protect employees who need to see clients alone. If you are in the situation of being entrusted to see clients on your own, it is essential that you ask your supervisor to help you clarify any parts of the placement policy that are unclear to you.

Personal safety

Generally speaking, your supervisors will forewarn you about any client who may present a threat while you are on placement. In any mental health setting it is impossible to always accurately predict the behaviour of some clients, especially during the assessment stage of their care. If you are with any client and your instinct tells you something is wrong – you feel at some sort of risk – then listen and react to this. Sometimes intuition is proved to be inaccurate, but sometimes it is right. If your 'gut feeling' is

telling you that there is danger, ignore any intellectual thoughts that argue things are alright. There are many simple things that you can do to minimise the risks that sometimes become present in mental health nursing:

- Tell colleagues where you are going with clients, and how long you are likely to be.
- Make sure they have heard you.
- Make sure you have your personal alarm with you.
- Make sure it works where you are going.
- Ensure you have an escape route open to you if you are in an enclosed area (e.g. sit or stand near an open door).
- Be aware of objects nearby that can be used to hurt you.
- Do not wear items of jewellery that could be used to hurt you (e.g. dangling earrings, scarves, necklaces).

Practice support from your university

If you feel you need additional support from your university tutors, do not hesitate to contact them. People come into the job of nursing from a wide diversity of cultures and experiences, and of course have a wide diversity of abilities. Most organisations that carry out nurse education have people within the organisation that can support this broad spectrum of need.

Many of your teachers and most of your mentors have come through a similar programme to the one that you are processing through. Additional support is not always directly linked to lesser ability. Given the diversity mentioned above, it is clear that every student nurse brings with them a history. For many, over the duration of the course, some aspect of their life will change. It is at these points that some students feel a need for extra support. It is probably best, as a generalisation, to ask for help sooner rather than later.

Switching off

Probably very difficult to do ... at first. This is because in some clinical settings the emotional stimulation within the area can be very intense. Even in low-activity areas, the very slow pace and the need to be 'doing something' can be a stress in itself.

Obvious ways to detach from the work environment usually involve diversion, although even the drive home can sometimes be done on 'automatic pilot' while you worry about what you should have said to that rude consultant, or difficult relative.

Most people are able to develop their own way of 'leaving work at work'. If this becomes difficult to manage then, informally, a trusted colleague may be able to help. A more organisationally formalised way is to contract to meet with a supportive supervisor, seen regularly or as and when required. This can be really helpful as a way of learning how to switch off, or disengage from work-related stress more effectively.

Making the most of insight visits

These should always be pre-arranged rather than impromptu. Try to be clear why it is that you want to carry out an insight visit. What specifically is it that you want to learn? Do some prereading about the speciality of the area first so that you are an informed visitor. Consolidate your visit with more reading or Internet searching. A very useful starting point for this, for example, is to search the Internet site for 'NICE Guidelines' appropriate for the area you wish to visit. This site is easy to access and will give you a good idea of some of the practicalities and dilemmas of care work in that type of placement.

It is often helpful to discuss the rationale for your visit to another placement area with your mentor. This can help to bring clarity to your objectives for the visit. In some instances these discussions lead to the creation of new placement opportunities as student visits can create or stimulate interest in the benefits that learners can bring to a clinical area. With this in mind, it is essential to be aware that when you undertake insight visits, you represent both your university and nursing students.

This concept of using your placement as a base, and 'outreaching' to other clinical settings, may become more predominant as a feature of future nurse training as the idea of the pathway placement model of organising placement sequencing is more widely adopted (see Ch. 4).

Finally, engage respectfully and sensitively with the people who work in your insight areas. You may want to revisit that area one day, as a prospective employee.

References

Archer, J., Wood, D.M., Tizzard, Z., Jones, A.L., Dargan, P.I., 2007. Alcohol hand rubs: hygiene and hazard. BMJ 335 (7630), 1154–1155.

Bairy, M., 2006. Bedside tipple?. Quality and Saftery in Health Care 15 (6), 446.

Batty, L., Brischetto, A., Kevat, A/C, Oldmeadow, M., 2011. Consumption of alcohol-based hand sanitisers by hospital inpatients. Medical Journal of Australia 194(12), 664.

Nursing and Midwifery Council, 2009. Guidance on professional conduct for nursing and midwifery students. NMC, London.

Further reading

Benner, P., 1984. From novice to expert: excellence and power in clinical nursing practice. Addison-Wesley, Menlo Park.

Clarke, V., Walsh, A., 2009. Fundamentals of mental health nursing. Oxford University Press, Oxford.

Norman, I., Ryrie, I., 2009. The art and science of mental health nursing. A textbook of principles and practice, 2nd ed. Open University Press, London.

Nursing and Midwifery Council, 2008. Supporting learning and assessment in practice. NMC, London.

Peters, T., Waterman, R., 2003. In search of excellence: lessons from America's best run companies. Profile Books, London.

Website

Nursing and Midwifery Council, http://www.nmc-uk.org.

Section 2. Practice-based learning and placement learning opportunities

The chapters within this section will aim to support you to develop the clinical skills which will enable you to respond effectively to mental health service users who are experiencing a range of problems and complex needs. The chapters will offer you a variety of approaches which you can adopt when working with people who use mental health services and aim to ensure your interventions are informed by a clear rationale and evidence base. While we view these skills as appropriate for a student mental health nurse to develop, it is important to discuss any planned interventions with your mentor before you attempt to apply them to your practice.

The section begins with broad skills which can be applied to any placement setting and moves on to explore skills which are suited to a specific difficulty the service user might be experiencing. It will finally look at the area of personal development. This will include exploring the attributes which will enable you to respond effectively to challenging situations in practice and how to begin to develop skills in leadership and management.

6 Broad skills for mental health nursing

CHAPTER AIMS

- To provide an outline of a range of broad skills utilised in various areas of mental health nursing practice
- To consider how these skills may be transferable to a range of settings

Introduction

This chapter aims to examine the techniques and skills in mental health nursing that lend themselves to working across any area and with any diagnosis. The following discussion considers the skills of communication, facilitating a group, solution-focused working and health promotion. The opportunity to develop these skills should be available in any placement area and will often provide the basis for meeting a substantial amount of your learning outcomes.

Communication skills in mental health settings

This section will explore an *intentioned, purposeful* and *effective* approach to communication as it can be used by mental health nurses in different clinical settings.

The application of this skill by nursing students will also be examined and discussed.

The first premise made in this section, as inferred above, is that there is something special about the skill of communication as used by effective nurses (Crawford et al 2006). This skill may sometimes be quite different from those used in non-work or social situations. This specialness is rooted in the nurse's 'intention' (Heron 2001) which originates in what the nurse is trying to achieve as part of care management.

Consider a community psychiatric nurse (CPN) calling at a service user's home for the first time to make an initial contact and assessment. The CPN will have a range of clear intentions. Some of these intentions will be clearly planned and obvious to an observer. Others may be reactive to the immediate situation, more subtle, not so easily detected and may even be such an integrated part of the nurse's professional personality that they are not aware of performing them until asked to reflect on what they are doing. For example, the skilled CPN is able to often process through a sufficiently comprehensive assessment of a service user, almost as if an everyday conversation is taking place (Bonham 2004). There is no sense of a 'cross-examination' or intrusive questioning. Areas of the service user's experience are examined and assessed with the minimum discomfort for the service user. At the same time, the nurse may sometimes be experiencing, at a deeper level, feelings or emotions which in a social context may be difficult (Bonham 2004). The experienced effective nurse develops the ability to manage these tensions by, for example, clinical supervision. Ask one of your mentors to give you illustrations of this.

The CPNs you work with may have more intentions, or a few less, than in the examples below, but you will see that the below sequence suggests a thoughtful, deliberate, intentional and strategic approach. This is very different from social interaction with friends, family, neighbours and so on, which is often more spontaneous, less considered and less goal or outcome orientated. The effective mental health nurse will therefore be constantly 'at work' within clinical areas. Some of this work may appear to be ordinary everyday conversation (Burnard 2003).

Consider this example. A mental health nurse is sitting with a service user in a secure rehabilitation unit. The nurse is wearing a uniform and has a highly visible personal alarm. Yet, to an outside observer, it looks as if the nurse and service user are at ease with each other. They could almost be friends having coffee together.

Activity

Review the list of intentions below with one of your mentors. Discuss which they routinely have, which they rarely have and which ones they have that are not listed. During interactions with service users, the CPN intends to:

- Create a climate of trust and approachability.
- Enable conversation to occur as naturally as possible.
- Keep the focus of the conversation with the service user.
- Explore issues being experienced by the service user.
- Listen intently to the language and delivery used by the service user.
- Support, validate and reassure the service user as appropriate.
- Do the above with any significant others who may be involved.
- Include any coworker (for example, you as a student).
- Limit questions that are asked to those which have a clear purpose.
- Encourage questions to be asked by the service user.
- Involve the service user in any plan of treatment.
- Be aware of timing, in terms of the needs of the service user, and other professional caseload demands.
- Clarify any issues which are unclear to the CPN, the service user or any other involved party, before finishing the visit.
- Leave the service user at least no more distressed, or anxious, than when the visit started, and possibly less so – if at all possible.
- Summarise any action or plan arising as a result of the visit.
- Confirm that the service user understands any action or plan.
- Confirm that the service user understands what is happening next, in terms of any input from the CPN or any other care professional who may be involved.
- Finish the visit at an appropriate point, and in a congruently positive way, if at all possible.

1. What are your impressions of this interaction?
2. What do you think might be the nurse's intention in this scenario?

Consider though ... this is not a social relationship. One person is a service user and one person is a professional receiving a salary. This is a professional being friendly, not a professional being a friend (Murray et al 1997, Jackson & Stevenson 1998). Just like the CPN above, the mental health nurse, in this quite different clinical environment, has a range of clear intentions which could be as follows:

- Be approachable (if you don't have this, how can you be effective?).
- Use social connectors such as a cup of tea, a newspaper, TV programmes, sport, plans for the day, and so on.
- Be aware of time constraints such as shift changes and meal times.
- Be aware of personal limitations – tiredness, other service users arranged to be seen during the shift, care plans to update, liaison with other professionals.
- Assess. How is the service user at this moment? Different from earlier today, yesterday, last week? If so, in what way?
- Edit. What is going to be added to the care plan as a result of this assessment?
- Be aware of anything that needs to be communicated to other colleagues – the service user is becoming increasingly agitated, the service user is more settled, etc.
- Create, sustain or finish a professional relationship.
- Maintain continuity – in terms of being clear to the service user that you will be back on duty tomorrow/next week/not at all.

Again it is clear that the nurse in this setting has some similar intentions, but some different intentions, from the CPN in the earlier example. Intention is, therefore, a function of the complexities of the clinical setting, the desired outcomes *of* the service user and *for* the service user, combined with the personality and desired outcomes of the nurse. This is perhaps why, despite having carried out what appear to be little more than a series of social interactions (but in a clinical setting), most effective mental health nurses find the work demanding and tiring, but also often very satisfying.

If the above range of intentions is examined more closely, they can be separated into identifiable skills. Most of these can be found in the body of literature on therapeutic interventions, communication skills, counselling and so on. This confirms the existence of a robust evidence base for the skills and attributes. These can be considered and discussed in the classroom, then practised in placement. As confidence and proficiency increase (this is a slow process for most people, by the way), the skills can be combined and blended into each other. They will become less conscious and more a part of your natural professional personality (Benner 1984).

Intention as separate communication skills and attributes 'Clusters'

Much of the literature on 'beginner' communication skills separates verbal from non-verbal skills. That separation will be apparent in the descriptions below, but you will also see how the two can be skilfully combined to form an effective, integrated whole. The following descriptors are the qualities you will see demonstrated by effective mental health nurses (and other mental health professionals) you will meet. They are not the raw communication skills you will see listed in most other texts. For instance, skills such as use of eye contact, touch, body positioning, voice tone and so on are discussed in the beginner literature. These areas will be discussed in classroom sessions during your time as a student nurse.

Activity

Discuss with your mentors how basic skills can be used to start to achieve the following more meaningful communication skills and attributes:

- Approachable
- Honest
- Encouraging clarity
- Consistent
- Transparent
- Optimistic
- Ordinary

- Knowledgeable
- Reliable
- Thoughtful
- Confident
- Empathic
- Assertive
- Accepting
- Use of language

- Pitch
- Eye contact
- Demeanour
- Touch
- Levels
- Proximity
- Tone of voce
- Gesture

Once you have considered basic separate skills, however, it is essential to refocus on the purpose of them and learn how to integrate them together.

Approachable

This is where it all starts (Bonham 2004). As a professional mental health nurse you are, in effect, being paid to be approachable. Other mental health professionals can use unapproachability to maintain distance between themselves and service users. It is a primary function of the mental health nurse to close that distance, professionally and skilfully. Not all service users wish to engage with mental health professionals, or even be friendly. If you are not sure what the individual components of approachability are, think about the colleagues you have met on placement. If you are just starting your career as a nurse, think of people you know who have this quality. What is it that seems to give them approachability? You'll find that the answer to this often lies in what they *do,* as much as in what they *say.* (Also consider – do you want to be approachable all the time?)

Honest

This personal characteristic is a good example of the difference between professionally outcome-driven strategic

 Activity

Consider with your mentor, or other students on your course, the skills cluster required to achieve approachability. Some components are the following:

- Suitably engaging eye contact (Egan 2002).
- A friendly or open demeanour (Bonham 2004).
- Professionally available body language.
- Manipulation of the environment, such as an open office door, or the deliberate positioning of oneself within the service user group rather than the professional group.
- Choice of clothing that suggests equality rather than superiority or striking difference, together with clarity of boundaries, i.e. the clarity has to be meaningful for the service user.

Identify with your mentor how you might demonstrate approachability and the opportunities which you might have to reflect and gain feedback on your approach.

communication as a skill, and social communication. In social situations you are at liberty to be deceitful, avoiding or open and direct to the point of brutality. You can 'call a spade a spade'.

In professional situations it is essential, for the safety and care of service users and your own professional credibility, that you are more considered and careful about what you say and how you say it. This pre-editing of your natural spontaneity can sometimes feel like avoidance or professional economy with the truth. The mental health nurse will often be in the situation of knowing more about certain issues than the service user. Often information is withheld from the service user as it is deemed to be '. . . in their best interests' (Nursing and Midwifery Council 2008). This view needs very careful consideration and must be the result of a multiprofessional consensus whenever realistically possible. Reflect with other students and your mentors on how to best manage these situations.

Encouraging clarity

This is a skill rather than a personal characteristic. As above, its use can be very different in professional situations compared to social situations.

( ) Reflection point

Consider this example:

A social setting . . .

Your friend: I hate this kind of situation.

You: Yeah. So do I.

A professional setting . . .

A service user: I hate this kind of situation.

You: What do you mean, you hate it?

1. What is the difference between the first example and the second?
2. How do you think the way you respond to the service user might impact on their reaction?

In the first example no effort is made to explore the nature of the word 'hate', the nature of the situation and the reasons for this view. In the second example the nurse has a strategy or intention to clarify. It may not be achieved immediately, during the next exchange, but the nurse is making a professional effort to *tentatively* (Bonham 2004) find out more, as part of a longer term assessing or monitoring, perhaps. It is important to note here that the above phrase 'What do you mean, you hate it?' can have many different impacts depending on how the words are delivered by the nurse. Try rehearsing some of these with another student and experiment with tone of voice, eye contact and general demeanour, to see the effect on the other person.

Consistent

Again, this aspect of communication can be very different in professional mental healthcare settings as compared with social situations. It does not mean 'sticking to your guns' regardless of changing circumstances around the care of the service user. The term means to be considered in your behaviour and attitude. These are two personality traits by which your effectiveness may be measured by service users and colleagues.

Both nurses in the examples above will be assessing, planning, implementing and evaluating the care they give (Norman & Ryrie 2009) as part of a consensus team approach. Even the CPN, who is more autonomous in terms of needing to make decisions about the care given, has to refer back to a team for support. That team will continue to give consistent, planned and agreed care. The original direction of this care may have come from the early meetings between the service user and the CPN. The team supports the carrying through of this care. So, to be consistent, the nurse must be empathic (Rogers 1951) to service users and colleagues, assertive with both, an effective listener to what is said and what is *not said* by both, sensitive to cultures and environments, a lateral thinker (de Bono 2009) and be open-minded to the ideas of others.

Transparent

Some other terms that can be linked to this are honesty, congruence, genuineness and authenticity (Rogers 1951). Like many of the attributes discussed in this section, transparency is not just something that is used in your interactions with service users. Some examples of transparent practice are the following:

• Fully including service users in all aspects of the management of their care, even the unpleasant or difficult ones, such as restricting their movements or unwanted adjustments to medication.
• Giving service users access to information written about them.

Just a little experience as a mental health nurse will tell you that the above examples of practice can sometimes be very difficult to carry through, and may actually have a negative effect on nurse–service user relationships. It can be difficult to judge an appropriate level of transparency when taking into account the immediate needs of a service user and the consequences of accessing or denying those needs. Transparency is something that is aspired to, but not always achieved.

Optimistic

Your work as a mental health nurse means that you are a professional optimist (Bonham 2004). In your personal life you may be pathologically pessimistic. In your professional life there is *always* hope for the service user you are working with. Looking at the caring role of the nurse at a very basic and pragmatic level, if you cannot visualise any hope for the service user you are working with then perhaps it is in the service user's best interests to minimise therapeutic contact with them. This might mean asking a colleague to take over the care of the person, referral to a

more suitable care agency, arranging clinical supervision to reflect with another how hope might be found or a team consensus may be to no longer engage with that person. An example of this is the person who continually self-harms despite, and regardless of, a range of therapeutic interventions by different concerned professionals. There may come a point when the input starts to become counterproductive. It may be more caring to withdraw support in a planned way, to try to foster independence, rather than dependence. This is in line with contemporary 'recovery' approaches (Repper & Perkins 2003) (see Ch. 3).

Ordinary

This is sometimes seen as a rather strange attribute for a mental health nurse – the ability to be ordinary or to possess ordinariness. It could be argued that this is a re-presentation of Rogers' core condition of congruence (or genuineness, honesty, authenticity). It is not. Ordinariness is a separate entity. To a large extent, within healthcare literature, clear references to ordinariness are few. The term is used in passing as the focus of the text is foregrounding something else. Occasionally it features in its own right as an attribute that some nurses have (Burnard 2003, Bonham 2004), and that is appreciated by service users. This does not just apply to mental health settings. Oblique reference to ordinariness can be found across the complete spectrum of health care (Dunniece & Slevin 2000, Blomqvist & Edberg 2002, Giske & Artinian 2007, Hopkins & Niemic 2007). To paraphrase these ideas, the nurse who has this therapeutic attribute can use their ordinariness to consolidate any stage of the therapeutic relationship. It can manifest itself in the following ways:

• Just 'being' with service users.
• Not necessarily needing to ask questions.
• Talking about self.

- Sharing food and drink.
- Being non-intrusive and consistently respectful of service users' space.

Knowledgeable

Even students who are at or near the end of their nursing course express the idea that they don't know enough to work effectively. Becoming deeply knowledgeable can only ever be a gradual process. Clinical experiences can accelerate and deepen knowledge in relatively narrow or specialised areas. For example, a mentor or a tutor with a particular interest or enthusiasm can help develop a focused knowledge within students. Thus, the nurse can become knowledgeable in the specific characteristics of the narcissistic personality disorder, but not know where the pharmacy is. Service users and colleagues usually do not expect even experienced staff to know everything. The key piece of knowledge for the student or newly qualified nurse is how to find out where the pharmacy is, what ward visiting hours are, when the consultant holds review meetings and so on, and then actually do it.

Reliable

Many student mental health nurses would probably consider this attribute as insignificant. Many mental health service users would probably think in a similar way. The time when reliability becomes most noticed by mental health nurses is when it is absent in a colleague. The time it is most noticed by the service user is when it is absent in a professional.

The nurse who is regularly absent from work, who is late for the start of a shift, who is missing from team meetings, can quickly become a liability to a team and may even become destructive to any sense of teamwork. The nurse who is often late for appointments with service users, or who has to regularly rearrange or miss meetings, quickly becomes the unwitting saboteur of any therapeutic relationship. The student nurse who often phones in sick, does not

phone in at all or has unplanned extra 'study days' becomes, in effect, an addition to the caseload of the mentor. Reliability is viewed as a 'given' in the range of essential mental health nurse attributes. Its absence is very noticeable and not appreciated.

Thoughtful

This could be remembering the names of people's significant others, of both service users and colleagues, or remembering meaningful dates and anniversaries. It could also mean being aware of colleagues who are having difficult lives outside of the work environment and facilitating adjustment to this if needed.

Confident

Most mental health nurses acquire this with accruing experience, accumulating knowledge and the passage of time. They start to feel more a part of a team or a culture. This really starts to happen once you become a qualified nurse and can settle into becoming part of a team, rather than a transient supernumerary person passing through. Queries can be answered without reference to a senior or more experienced colleague. Difficult situations can be managed by leading rather than following. This process can be constructively accelerated by using clinical supervision, self-reflection, peer reflection and so on.

Empathic

The often quoted understanding of the quality of being empathic, or demonstrating empathy, is to have the ability to '... get inside the service user's world and experience their thoughts and feelings in that world ...' (Clarke & Walsh 2009). It is definitely *not* about having had the same experience as someone else. It is more about having the ability, or at least willingness, to try to get a sense of what the other person is experiencing now, has experienced in the past or may experience in the future. An essential characteristic of being empathic is the verbalisation of this sense. It is no use to the service user if you are thinking to yourself as they describe their problems: 'That must have been pretty difficult for them.'

An example of how the service user could be included would be:

Service user: It was then I told her that I couldn't put up with her behaviour any longer . . . so she left.

Nurse: That must have been pretty difficult for you?

Service user response 1: Yes it got really bad then. I didn't know what to do with myself. I felt terrible.
  or

Service user response 2: No. Actually it was a relief. At last I'd said it to her. I felt good for a while.
  or

Service user response 3: Well . . . in some ways, yes. I was alone again. But that was OK.

Notice that in 'Service user response 1' the nurse has been effectively empathic. She has focused on the difficulty of the situation by thinking about how she might have felt in a similar situation to the service user. In this instance the service user responds by confirming that the nurse's thoughts are appropriate (or near enough). This shows the service user that the nurse has been listening and is, at that moment, 'tuned in' to the service user. The nurse's verbal response is a clear example of 'active listening', i.e. there is a clear *active* response by the nurse. Notice the carefully questioning tone of the nurse's intervention. She is being appropriately tentative, and not overconfident. This is a sustaining attitude to have, in terms of keeping a therapeutic relationship productive.

In 'Service user response 2' it looks at first as if the nurse has got it wrong. You will note, though, that the service user gives a new piece of information to the nurse. The

story has changed direction, but the nurse's initially misdirected attempt to empathise is the catalyst for this.

In 'Service user response 3', again, it looks as if the empathic intention has missed the mark. If you examine the service user's response, however, you can see that again it contains ideas from which the therapeutic dialogue can be usefully developed further. As long as you are thoughtful and careful, your attempts at empathy may not always be accurate, but they will more often than not be useful in terms of advancing the therapeutic process.

Assertive

This is not about always getting your own way. It is important to realise that the job you are training to do will involve you in conflict of some form at some time. The effective nurse will learn when to avoid conflict and when to become involved in it. The conflict may be with any other person you encounter during your working day. It can be with service users, psychiatrists, social workers . . . anyone. Conflict will be caused by issues from the differing views of what is in the service users' 'best interests' through to the territorial behaviours of healthcare professionals. The nurse can be the unwitting catalyst of this conflict trying to advocate for a service user, for example. Or she may find herself acting as the mediator between a social worker and a relative of the service user.

The effectively assertive nurse will be able to listen to a range of views with a relatively detached degree of objectivity (Bonham 2004). They will have the skills to paraphrase and summarise the views of themselves and others (Bonham 2004). They will be aware of body language – both controlling their own and reading that of others.

Accepting

This is an ability rather than a skill. The term may be seen, in other texts, as 'non-judgemental', possessing 'unconditional positive regard' (Rogers 1951). It means that the effective mental health nurse can meet with and interact with any person that she meets professionally, and leave her own values, attitudes and beliefs outside the assessment and treatment of the service user's issues. The evidence of this can be seen in a consistent, considered and measured approach to all service users, regardless of the history they bring with them.

Use of language

The confusion caused by misunderstanding language and consequential inappropriate or poor treatment has a long history in all forms of nursing and especially mental health nursing where culture and nuance of language are pivotal in assessing and treating accurately.

(|) **Reflection point**

Consider these examples:

- I hate it here.
- I hate tea with sugar in.
- I hate it when you're like this.
- I hate that consultant.
- I hate this medication.
- I love this place.
- I love you.
- I love fish and chips.
- I love the summer.
- I love Tiddles.

Think about the countless ways in which these few words can be delivered to you as a student nurse by people of different:

1. ages
2. cultures
3. genders.

What might be the implications of this and how might you ensure that you ascertain the right meaning for that individual?

The meaning of each of the above statements will differ according to who is saying it and the manner in which they express it, be that speaking, whispering, shouting, writing or texting. It is part of your job as a mental health nurse to be consistently reliable and accurate in your understanding of what people mean, and transfer some or all of that information verbally and/or in writing to your professional colleagues appropriately while at the same time taking into account issues such as confidentiality, privacy and dignity. The student nurse whose first language is not English may need extra support from their tutorial staff and clinical mentors.

Pitch

This is the skill of being able to account for or compensate for the diversity in communication, language and intellectual abilities that mental healthcare management will present to you. Consider how you alter your 'pitch' to communicate effectively with a terrified Iranian asylum seeker who has been admitted to your ward as compared to the pitch you use with the teenage son of a woman suffering with psychotic symptoms who you visit in her own home.

Non-verbal presentation of the above
Eye contact

There is no such thing as 'good' eye contact. The effective nurse uses *appropriate* eye contact depending on the situation presenting. Sometimes this can mean very little eye contact, or even no eye contact. Discuss with your mentors how this could be true.

Demeanour

Positive, approachable, relaxed, respectful, at ease with oneself – these are ideal components of a therapeutic demeanour.

Touch

This is a very potent means of communicating quickly and deeply with someone, but its use needs a considered approach. To use touch spontaneously can have a mixed result. Its effect can be welcomed by the person being touched. It can be very comforting. On the other hand, it can be received as offensive and distancing. It is to be used with great care.

Levels

Consider how you might best communicate with a confused and frightened female service user of 85 years old, as compared with a 9-year-old male service user. Should you be using your body language to help you work more effectively? If a child is playing on the floor it might be most effective, in terms of connecting with them, to sit in the floor at the same level. There is no clear rule for this kind of situation. It is clear, though, that consideration of issues like this makes a great difference to communication channels.

Proximity

Similarly, how near should you position yourself to service users? Should you be across the room, or close enough to touch them? Your proximity will make a considerable impact on the effectiveness of your interaction. Variables such as the clinical setting and relationship with the service user will help decide the optimum positioning you should take to maximise your effectiveness. Discuss how proxemics are considered in clinical practice with your mentors.

Tone of voice

A hard tone of voice may be distancing. A soft tone may be patronising. The tone is one of the key factors that govern how a spoken message is received.

Gesture

Do you 'windmill' your hands around or keep them in your pocket when talking with others as a professional? As above, it is useful to reflect on this with other students and mentors, specifically how hand movement can sometimes help, or sometimes distract, from the effectiveness of a professional interaction.

Self-awareness

Why it matters

Self-awareness is important because, as part of your job, it is essential that you maximise the effectiveness of your communication with others. This is particularly important in the field of mental health nursing as so much of the job is communication, using voice, body language, telephone and writing. In all these media you present a version of yourself that gives others an impression of what you are like as a person, and what your intentions are as a professional. It is important, therefore, that you manage the image that you present. Poor or inaccurate awareness of yourself means that this can be a very hit-and-miss process.

Impact on others

Even as a student nurse you have the potential to significantly alter a person's experience as a patient. Remember what it is like for you to be waiting in a room in a strange environment with people who work there coming and going without acknowledging you, or letting you know what is happening. It can make a huge difference to a person's experience by taking the trouble to just let them know that: 'The doctor has been delayed on another call ... she'll be about another 30 minutes. I'll let her know that you've arrived'.

The way that these few words are delivered by you are highly significant in terms of the effect they can have on the recipient. Say the above sentence with different tones of voice, or with a smile then a frown. Imagine the different impact you can have with these changes.

How you gain it

You look for it – in the reactions of others towards you. How do others react to you? Are they calmer, more agitated, indifferent? You acquire it by copying the good practices of the other professionals around you, and by not repeating or colluding in the poorer practices you might see. As a student you are in the perfect position to ask for feedback from your mentors and supervisors as part of your professional development.

Social self-awareness and professional self-awareness

These two aspects of you are different. As mentioned above, the most significant difference is that you are being paid to be effective and efficient at being a nurse. When you are on duty you represent the organisation that pays you. Your customers (patients/clients/service users/residents/other professionals/general public) are entitled to a professional, respectful, efficient service from you as a mental health nurse. This is regardless of the stage of training or career you are at, or the clinical setting.

Off duty, people will still have expectations of you because of the traditions of the job you are training for. In some respects, then, the need to be aware of self carries on after you leave your area of work.

> **◐ Reflection point**
>
> One way of enhancing your self-awareness is to critically question yourself on assumptions or decisions you have made. For example, when people ask you why you wanted to become a nurse you may respond with something like 'I enjoy working with people'. If you ask yourself this question again you may have a different response which you wouldn't necessarily want to share with others but that you are aware influenced your decision. For example, you may have a family member who experiences mental health problems which has led you to be interested in helping others. Take some time to ask yourself this question and reflect upon how this might influence the way you practise as a nurse.

Solution-focused brief therapy

Solution-focused work has its origins within psychological approaches. It emerged in the 1970s, influenced by the work of key psychologists at the time. It was in the 1980s that it developed as a more defined therapeutic approach through the work of de Shazer and colleagues (de Shazer 1985, de Shazer et al 1986). The main premise of solution-focused therapy is that therapeutic gains (which are defined by the person using the service) can be achieved by concentrating on what the individual *can* do and what they want to achieve. Focusing entirely on problems and difficulties of the past are therefore seen as inhibiting the creation of positive changes for the future. Solution-focused work is a form of therapy where individuals can undertake specialist training. It is also designed as a 'brief' intervention so the number of sessions between an individual and therapist are minimal. However, it is a therapeutic technique which can be incorporated into the interpersonal work of a mental health nurse, particularly as it shares its underlying principles with the strengths model and recovery approach. There is an increasing amount of literature which examines its potential for nursing practice (McAllister 2007, Wand 2010).

The underpinning philosophy of solution-focused therapy is based on the view that the service users are the experts and that they are able to define their own solutions and set their own goals (Ferraz & Wellman 2009). Potentially this is quite a shift away from the traditional manner in which health professionals work. We are used to identifying and assessing problems and offering our expertise on a solution to this problem. Indeed, when first using solution-focused techniques it can feel quite alien. Yet, recognising the expertise offered by service users is important. Solution-focused techniques also offer a very practical application of the principles of the strengths model and recovery approach.

Questions which are solution orientated are employed to identify what the person perceives is working in their lives rather than what isn't. This enables the service user and the worker to focus on how solutions are developed and constructed, therefore creating positive change (Hanton 2009).

Solution-focused questions to elicit goals might include:

- What are you hoping to get from us working together?
- How will you know the work has been successful?
- How will other people know that things are better?

It is important to recognise that the solution that the person proposes might not reflect the problem that professionals have identified that needs working on. For instance, someone might identify that they would know the work has been successful because they are being a supportive sister or they have started Karaoke again. These roles and interests may have become invisible within the difficulties and problems that their contact with health services has brought focus on. Accepting this difference

in perceived priorities is part of the nurse recognising the expertise and experience that the individual brings, which is so significant within a solution-focused approach.

Such a form of enquiry also asks the individual to think about their preferred future and positive coping resources. This provides an opportunity to explore in depth how they might want their future to look different, moving beyond the problems they are currently facing (Ferraz & Wellman 2009, Hanton 2009). One of the main ways that this is addressed is by asking the 'miracle question'. Framing this question may feel a little odd initially, for both the service user and the worker, particularly as it is so different from how we usually approach problems. It would be fine to acknowledge this at the start.

Miracle question

Imagine if you were to go to sleep tonight and you woke up tomorrow morning and a miracle had occurred. This miracle was that all the problems that were concerning you have been solved. However, because it took place while you were asleep you didn't know that the miracle had happened. What is the first thing that you would notice in the morning that would tell you the miracle has happened (de Shazer 1988)?

Using the miracle question provides an opening for a miracle and solution-focused conversation to take place (Wand 2010). This entails involving the individual in visualising and imagining the changes that the miracle would create in depth. Therefore, the miracle question may be followed by further questions such as:

- How would your husband/mother/ partner know that the miracle has occurred?
- What is the first thing that they would notice?
- What will you be doing differently when the miracle happens?

- What is it that will be different when you are smiling more/talking to your brother/ feeling happier?

This miracle dialogue can then be followed with asking the individual whether they have noticed any small part of the miracle taking place, exploring, therefore, their current achievements and resources as part of this process. Scaling questions are a really useful tool employed within the solution-focused approach. These can help break down what may seem overwhelming and out of reach into smaller, more manageable, chunks.

Scaling questions include:

- On a scale of 1 to 10, with 1 being the absolute worst it can ever be and 10 being you are on top of things, where are you today ?
- Ok ... you are a 2 today. What stops you being a 1?
- What would it look like if you were a 3?
- What would it take to reach a 3?

Wand (2010) also provides some useful examples of how these kinds of questions may be used for someone who may be feeling suicidal. Solution-focused interventions consider that there are always exceptions, so look at times when the problem didn't occur or times when it wasn't as bad as the person expected. Exploring these exceptions is important, particularly when it can be difficult for the individual to identify positives, resources and coping. This enables them to consider a situation more optimistically.

The example below puts together the techniques examined here to provide an insight into how a solution-focused conversation may be conducted, picking up the conversation after the miracle question has been asked:

Nurse–service user interaction

Nurse: So what would be the first thing that you noticed in the morning that would tell you the miracle has happened?

Person: Well, I don't know ... I suppose that the weight from my chest and the tightness in my head wasn't there any more.

Nurse: How will you know that the weight from your chest and the tightness in your head wasn't there anymore?

Person: I suppose I might be able to sit up straight away.

Nurse: What else ...?

Person: I would be able to breathe and ... I don't know, maybe it might change the way I feel about facing the day.

Nurse: Ok ... that sounds important, so what might you be doing that would show that you felt you could face the day?

Person: Well ... I would take a shower and then go and make James a cup of coffee.

Nurse: You would make James a cup of coffee; so how else might James know the miracle had happened?

Person: Well ... maybe he would see that I was happier ...

Nurse: So what would you be doing that would show that you are happier?

Person: I don't know, I'd be able to get out of bed and ... then ... then plant those vegetables in the garden that I've always wanted to and, I don't know, it sounds silly but I'd be smiling!

Nurse: That's not silly. So on a scale of 1 to 10 with 1 being the most unhappy you have been and 10 being happy, 10 being the vegetables have been planted in the garden ... where would you put yourself on that scale today?

Person: Maybe about a 3.

Nurse: About a 3 ... so what stops you being a 2.

Person: Well I am here. If I was a 2, I don't think I would have been able to get here. If I was a 2, the tightness in my head would have been too much to get in the car, but with a 3 it is a bit better; it fades enough for me to get out which is good.

Nurse: So what will it be like when you reach 4?

Person: I don't know ... I think at a 4, I think I would perhaps ... I would have a bit more energy, perhaps be able to do the washing before coming here.

Nurse: How will you know that you have reached 4? What will James notice?

As you can see, one of the important aspects of using a solution-focused technique is adopting the language that is used by the individual. It also entails accepting possibilities. You'll notice that the words used by the nurse assume that these changes will be made and reached (e.g. what will it look like when you reach 4?).

This section has provided an overview of a solution-focused approach and introduced some tools that could be incorporated into practice with individuals within a variety of mental health practice settings.

Facilitating groups

Facilitating a group for therapeutic purposes can be a really valuable way to offer support. Groups developed with this aim are common within mental health services and can be facilitated by many different workers. Self-help and peer support groups can also be particularly powerful. Examples of this might include those developed and run by the Hearing Voices Network to offer support for people who hear voices.

Facilitating a group offers a number of benefits which include the following:

- The expertise and experience of others in the group.
- Giving and receiving peer support.

- Learning from one another, sharing experiences.
- Cohesiveness – being part of a close group.
- Sharing a sense of 'we are all in this together'.
- Cost-effectiveness and resources – providing support/interventions/ education to a number of people at one time.

However, there are also some difficulties and limitations associated with facilitating a group:

- Relations within groups can be complex and difficult dynamics might arise, which can be stressful to experience and manage.
- Not all groups make full use of their members effectively – some people may dominate or not participate fully.
- It could lead to difficulty with decision making.

Groups are naturally occurring within society and have been described as important for the functioning of humanity. They can offer social and psychological benefits in terms of identify, self-esteem and wellbeing (Barker 2003). Setting up and running a group can therefore be a useful way to provide and enable support for people experiencing mental distress. There are various areas where running a group may be particularly helpful, but common groups facilitated by mental health nurses include anxiety management, recovery and 'hearing voices' groups.

Setting up a group

Before starting a group, it is important to consider an aim for the group. This helps to give an outline of its purpose. It provides an opportunity to think about potential outcomes for group members, although this is something that could also be done in collaboration with group members during the early stages of a group forming.

Recognising the purpose of a group and the reason for setting it up helps to provide structure and answer some key questions that need to be considered when establishing a group, such as:

- How long will it run?
- What is an optimum or appropriate group size?
- Will membership change and can people join at different stages?
- Where is the best place for it to be located?

Some groups grow more organically and their purpose might change as the group evolves. They may have a more informal structure such as a social or art group. However, it is useful to identify these aims in planning a group to help all those who attend get the most out of it as well as helping to identify any potential challenges or problems.

Some groups can benefit from structure. This entails more planning and will involve considering the aim or plan for each week. For instance, a 'hearing voices' group may be focused around understanding and interpretation of voices one week, and another around sharing ways that people cope with voices. The facilitators could plan key questions that they may ask members to encourage discussion, or exercises they might do to provide information in an interesting way.

Running a group

It can help to have some basic guidelines to help manage relationships within a group, set clear expectations from the start and establish boundaries. This, again, is best achieved in collaboration with the whole group at the start of the group forming. These might include the following issues:

- Respect and listening – ensuring all have an opportunity to contribute.
- Confidentiality – what is kept in the group and what can be or has to be shared outside the group.

- Arrangements – such as punctuality, plans for meeting location if group is social, what people will bring (if needed).

The facilitator's role

The role of the group facilitator will vary depending on the nature of the group. Some groups will involve providing education which may require the facilitator to take on a more directive role at points during the process. There are a number of core features that define the role of a facilitator and contribute to a cohesive and effective group.

A facilitator does not lead a group through telling; they should guide rather than direct a group. This might involve the following:

- Not answering all questions themselves but returning this to the group for discussion.
- Enabling participation of all group members; at times asking some to listen and allow others to contribute alongside inviting quieter members to have their say.
- Stepping back and encouraging groups to make decisions for themselves.
- Reminding members of the aims and guidelines agreed at the start of the group if necessary.

Through these mechanisms, a facilitator can help create a safe and welcoming space in which people can be open and the group can come together.

Ending a group

The end of the group is as important as the preceding stages. Plans need to be made about how a group is to finish (for groups that are ongoing, remember changes in members or functions might represent the ending of one group and the beginning of another). This will entail agreeing an expected timeline and processing any outstanding issues through discussion as a group. Such a process is aimed at ensuring that there are not any unresolved conflicts

Table 6.1 Lifecycle of a group

Stage	Characteristics
Forming	Entails examining what the group is supposed to be doing and how the group works Members will try to create a good impression of themselves They are more likely to seek direction and help from the facilitators
Storming	Conflicts and disagreements within the group are common This can create challenges to power and boundaries These might be shown through not coming to the group or arriving late
Norming	The group feels more comfortable with each other and group rules/norms are clearly established
Performing	The group functions as a whole, they work together well and are productive
Mourning	The group comes to an end so adjustments need to be made to loss and change

relating to the group that members are left with. Chapter 7 deals with the ending of therapeutic relationships which will help provide some tips for how this may be approached. On a practical note, finishing would include summarising what the group has achieved and helping members make action plans about how they will take this forward.

Tuckman (1965) provides a model to outline the lifecycle of a group which can aid in reflecting on the group process (see Table 6.1). This reflects the stages that a group is likely to go through and may help you understand changes in the functioning of a group that you may be facilitating or a part of (such as the group you are a part of for the theoretical component of your course).

Group dynamics

A psychodynamic perspective on groups suggests that interpersonal relations are formed and people learn about themselves in relation to others through the group process. Relating to others within a group situation creates the potential for tension and dynamics to result at times from the

way the individuals in the group relate to one another. Group dynamics refers to the way a group functions. Dynamics can be affected by a number of aspects which include the following:

• The individual characteristics of the members.
• The group qualities in terms of values, communication, size, how cohesive the group is.
• The task – how stressful it is, norms and consequences.
• Structures such as roles that people adopt within the group and power relations.

Agreeing guidelines at the start of the group process which can be revisited can be helpful in managing some dynamics. Exploring dynamics within your own supervision (ensuring agreed confidentiality is maintained) is important for a facilitator to help manage relations and help promote optimum functioning within the group.

This section has provided an insight into some of the key areas to think about when planning, implementing and ending a therapeutic group. Chapter 8 focuses on interpersonal skills and may aid in helping to put some of these skills into practice.

Health promotion

Mental health promotion became a key element of the mental health nurses' role with the publication of the *National Service Framework for Mental Health* (Department of Health 1999). This document emphasised the roles and responsibilities of mental health practitioners in this area of practice and stated that health and social services should:

1. Promote mental health for all, working with individuals and communities.
2. Combat discrimination against individuals and groups with mental health problems and promote their social inclusion.

This can involve a range of activities focused on how individuals, families, organisations and communities think and feel and the factors which influence this individually and collectively. It also acknowledges the impact that mental wellbeing has on overall health and the cohesiveness of communities. This involves looking at the impact of the social environment on health and addressing the link between disease patterns and the way in which society is organised.

The examples in Tables 6.2 and 6.3 illustrate how your practice can enhance mental health and tackle some of the factors which challenge mental health. These are informed by Albee and Ryan Finn's (1993) 10 elements of mental health promotion

Table 6.2 Promoting the physical health of people with mental health problems

Level	Example
Micro	Julia has high blood pressure and is overweight. The mental health practitioner works with her to give her information on the impact of her weight on her physical health and explores how her appearance influences her confidence and self-esteem. She identifies that a key barrier for her in addressing the problem is the way she is treated at the local swimming pool. She feels that staff are rude to her and discourage her from using the pool because they think she is crazy and will hurt other people
Meso	The mental health practitioner makes an appointment with the manager of the swimming pool to consider ways of addressing this problem. When Julia and the mental health practitioner meet with him they are surprised at his attitude towards people with mental health problems and recognise that this is informed by a lack of accurate information and concern about how to respond to people if they get distressed while using the facilities. The mental health practitioner offers to run a series of sessions with the swimming pool staff to give them information and look at how they might support a person in distress. Julia offers to share her experiences with the staff and talk about what she finds helpful in supporting her to access community services
Macro	The mental health practitioner writes to the council to inform them of the intervention and discuss how this could be rolled out across the area

Table 6.3 Maintaining employment

Level	Example
Micro	The mental health practitioner is working with Darren who has a diagnosis of obsessional compulsive disorder (OCD). At work, Darren washes his hands up to 40 times a day. He is aware that his colleagues have recognised his problems and suspects that they ridicule him behind his back. His manager has issued him with a formal warning as a result of the impact that his handwashing is having on his quality of work. He feels isolated, stressed and is seriously considering quitting his job. The mental health practitioner works with Darren to first explore the impact of his environment on his mental wellbeing and identify that his handwashing is exacerbated by his colleagues' attitudes. The mental health practitioner considers alternative ways of coping with his anxiety at work and approaches to addressing his colleagues' attitude towards him. He also supports Darren to inform his manager of his mental health problem and challenge his formal warning
Meso	The mental health practitioner is told by Darren that his manager was not interested to hear about his problems and maintains that if he can't do the job then he needs to be penalised irrelevant of the circumstances. With Darren's permission, the practitioner contacts the manager to discuss with him the Disability Discrimination Act (1995). The manager is not aware that the Act includes people with mental health problems and has assumed it only applied to people with physical disabilities. He tells the mental health practitioner that he will retract Darren's formal warning and also inform other line managers in the company to ensure that they do not make a similar mistake
Macro	The mental health practitioner writes a letter to a national newspaper reporting on the concern about the potential for large companies to fail to understand and apply the Disability Discrimination Act (1995). The letter is published and they receive a number of responses thanking them for drawing attention to this problem and telling them about similar experiences

and demotion. This model identifies that impact can be made at the micro (individual), meso (community) and macro (policy and legislation) levels. In order to promote mental health, interventions should be focused on enhancing the areas of environmental quality, self-esteem, emotional processing, self-management skills and social participation or, alternatively, minimising the impact of environment deprivation, emotional abuse, emotional negligence, stress and social exclusion.

⟨•⟩ Reflection point

For the examples above:
1. Identify the factors which promote or demote mental health.
2. Identify the interventions put in place by the mental health practitioner at each of the levels.
3. In your placement area, think about activities which you have observed, or been involved in, which promote an individual's mental health. Consider how you might apply this at a meso or macro level.

The examples above demonstrate how the individual practitioner can influence perceptions of mental health problems at all levels through simple interventions which educate, inform and challenge stigma and discrimination. It may feel at times that negative attitudes towards people with mental health problems is entrenched, however evidence supports the impact of interventions such as these and emphasises the importance of mental health practitioners taking an active stance towards this social issue.

References

Albee, G.W., Ryan Finn, K.D., 1993. An overview of primary prevention. Journal of Counselling and Development 72 (2), 115–123.

Barker, P., 2003. Psychiatric and mental health nursing: the craft of caring. Hodder and Arnold, London.

Benner, P., 1984. From novice to expert: excellence and power in clinical nursing practice. Addison–Wesley, Menlo Park.

Blomqvist, K., Edberg, A., 2002. Older people living with persistent pain. Journal of Advanced Nursing 40 (3), 297–306.

Bonham, P., 2004. Communicating as a mental health carer. Nelson Thornes, Cheltenham.

Burnard, P., 2003. Ordinary chat and therapeutic conversation: phatic communication and mental health nursing. Journal of Psychiatric and Mental Health Nursing 10 (6), 678–682.

Clarke, V., Walsh, A., 2009. Fundamentals of mental health nursing. Oxford University Press, Oxford.

Crawford, P., Brown, B., Bonham, P., 2006. Communication in clinical settings. Nelson Thornes, Cheltenham.

de Bono, E., 2009. Lateral thinking: a textbook of creativity. Penguin, London.

de Shazer, S., 1985. Keys to solutions in brief therapy. Norton, New York.

de Shazer, S., 1988. Clues: investigating solutions in brief therapy. Norton, New York.

de Shazer, S., Berg, I.K., Lipchick, E., et al., 1986. Brief therapy: focused solution development. Family Process 25 (2), 207–221.

Department of Health, 1999. National Service framework for mental health: modern standards and service models. HMSO, London.

Dunniece, U., Slevin, E., 2000. Nurses' experience of being present with a service user receiving a diagnosis of cancer. Journal of Advanced Nursing 32 (3), 603–610.

Egan, G., 2002. The skilled helper, 7th ed. Brookes Cole, Pacific Grove.

Ferraz, H., Wellman, N., 2009. Fostering a culture of engagement; an evaluation of a 2 day training in solution focused brief therapy for mental health workers. Journal of Psychiatric and Mental Health Nursing 16, 326–334.

Giske, T., Artinian, B., 2007. Patterns of 'balancing between hope and despair' in the diagnostic phase: a grounded theory study of service users on a gastroenterology ward. Journal of Advanced Nursing 62 (1), 22–31.

Hanton, P., 2009. Solution focused therapy in a problem focused world. Healthcare Counselling and Psychotherapy Journal 9 (2).

Heron, J., 2001. Helping the service user, 5th ed. Sage, London.

Hopkins, C., Niemic, S., 2007. Mental health crisis at home: service user perspectives on what helps and what hinders. Journal of Psychiatric and Mental Health Nursing 14, 310–318.

Jackson, S., Stevenson, C., 1998. The gift of time from the friendly professional. Nursing Standard 12 (51), 31–33.

McAllister, M., 2007. Solution focused nursing; rethinking practice. Palgrave McMillan, Basingstoke.

Murray, A., Shepherd, G., Onyett, S., Muijen, M., 1997. More than a friend. Sainsbury Centre for Mental Health, London.

Norman, I., Ryrie, I., 2009. The art and science of mental health nursing. A textbook of principles and practice, 2nd ed. Open University Press, London.

Nursing and Midwifery Council, 2008. The code: standards of conduct, performance and ethics for nurses and midwives. NMC, London.

Repper, J., Perkins, R., 2003. Social inclusion and recovery: a model for mental health practice. Baillière Tindall, Oxford.

Rogers, C., 1951. Service user centred therapy. Houghton Mifflin, Boston.

Tuckman, B.W., 1965. Developmental sequence in small groups. Psychological Bulletin 63 (6), 384–399.

Wand, T., 2010. Mental health nursing from a solution focused perspective. International Journal of Mental Health Nursing 19, 210–219.

Further reading

Bonham, P., 2004. Communicating as a mental health carer. Nelson Thornes, Cheltenham.

Stickley, T., Stacey, G., 2009. Caring: the essence of mental health nursing. In: Callaghan, P., Playle, J., Cooper, L. (Eds.), Mental health nursing skills. Oxford University Press, Oxford.

7

Forming, maintaining and ending therapeutic relationships

CHAPTER AIMS

- To identify the theory and evidence that underpin the importance of the therapeutic relationship in mental health practice
- To consider the skills and attributes that facilitate the development and maintenance of the therapeutic relationship
- To discuss the challenges and complexities present at various stages of the therapeutic relationship

Introduction

The concept of the therapeutic relationship is central to mental health nursing practice. It enables the provision of nursing care through engagement and delivery of specific clinical skills such as assessment, care planning, intervention and supporting the person to move on from mental health services. Despite the central position of the therapeutic relationship within mental health nursing, it is often difficult to define or identify exactly what it looks like in practice. Aldridge (2006) acknowledges that it is due to its complexity and the level of skill required to develop this aspect of

practice. Definitions often imply it is a purposeful human interaction that has a specific intent or goal aimed at meeting a service user's needs or best interests. It is based upon building a genuine human alliance which enables collaborative approaches to practice (Barker & Buchanan-Barker 2005). It may be a brief interaction or a relationship that spans over several years.

This chapter will explore and apply the theories that underpin the rationale for the importance of the therapeutic relationship, and consider approaches which may be helpful to you in your practice when developing skills which facilitate the forming, maintaining and ending of therapeutic relationships.

As a student mental health nurse you will have the opportunity to spend a great deal of time with people who are using mental health services. This will provide you with the opportunity to begin to develop these skills right from the beginning of your journey to becoming a qualified nurse.

Underpinning theory

The concept of the therapeutic relationship is largely related to the work of Carl Rodgers (1951) and person-centred approaches. Rodgers maintains that therapeutic relationships should be underpinned by core conditions which are conducive to emotional growth and wellbeing. These include genuineness or congruence, unconditional positive regard and empathy.

Genuineness or congruence

This refers to being honest within the relationship and being open to offering some of yourself in order for the person to recognise you as human and not just as a professional.

Consider the following situations:

1. You are working with a service user who is having difficulties with her daughter coming home late and not wanting to get up for school. This is having a negative effect on their relationship and leading to daily arguments. You tell the service user that you also have a daughter of a similar age who is behaving in a similar way. You disclose that you are also finding it hard to deal with and share her concerns about how it is affecting your relationship with your daughter.

2. You are working with a service user who continuously attempts to kiss or hug you during every interaction. You find yourself wanting to avoid him as it makes you feel uncomfortable. You arrange a one-to-one session with the service user and explain how it makes you feel when he approaches you in this way. You clarify that you do want to spend time with him but that his behaviour makes you feel uncomfortable and is not appropriate within a professional relationship.

◖◗ Reflection point

1. How have you demonstrated genuineness within these scenarios?
2. What might be challenging about demonstrating this level of honesty within the therapeutic relationship?
3. How might you manage these challenges?

Unconditional positive regard

This describes the ability to see beyond a person's behaviour to recognise them as an individual. This requires you to be aware of your prejudgements and have the willingness to show absolute acceptance.

Consider the following examples below:

1. You are working with a service user who tells you that she is using illicit drugs while she is pregnant. She is aware of the harm she may be doing to her unborn baby but is not able to stop. You explore with her the reasons why she continues to take the drugs and identify that it provides her with escapism from the memories of a prior abusive and violent relationship. This enables you to understand her behaviour and work with her to consider other ways of responding to her distress. You let her know that her drug taking is understandable but that she does have other options.

◖◗ Reflection point

1. What is your initial reaction when you read that a service user is using drugs while pregnant?
2. How might you explore your reaction in order to enable you to work with the service user effectively?
3. What might be the challenge of doing so?

2. You have been working with a service user for a number of months to support him to move on from the residential rehabilitation unit. Other members of the team are sceptical that he will go through with the move as he has reached this stage in the past but has then engaged in behaviour which the team describes as sabotaging his move. Despite this view, you maintain a positive attitude towards him and reiterate your belief in his potential to live independently.

1. How might you maintain this positive attitude when others are sceptical?
2. Why is it important that you maintain your belief in the service user as opposed to agreeing with the other members of the team?

Empathy

This refers to being able to see the world from the view of another person in order to experience their thoughts and feelings. This allows you to explore how their thoughts and feelings might influence their actions and behaviours.

Think about the examples in the scenarios above.

1. Identify the elements of the examples which show how empathy towards the service user has been demonstrated.
2. Consider how you may feel if you were working with the service users described here.
3. What might influence your reaction and response?
4. What might challenge you in demonstrating empathy towards the person?
5. How might you work around this in order to provide the core conditions of the therapeutic relationship?

Forming therapeutic relationships

It is often assumed that the formation of therapeutic relationships is inevitable and that service users should automatically trust a healthcare practitioner due to their role and title. This is often not the case in mental health services for a number of reasons:

- The person may not agree that they have a mental health problem and therefore do not require your support. This is sometimes referred to as lacking insight.
- The person may have had negative experiences in the past with mental health practitioners or other people they perceive as having authority and therefore are sceptical or suspicious about your intentions.
- The person may have found previous contact with mental health services traumatic.
- The person may be concerned about the stigma associated with being involved with mental health services and therefore reluctant to have any association with you.
- The person may be fearful that they will be forced to make changes to their lifestyle which they do not want to alter.
- The person may have been advised by their community not to have contact with mental health services due to their cultural or religious beliefs about mental health problems and their perception of Western service and treatments.
- The person may be sceptical about the value of your involvement and have little faith in your ability to make a difference to their distress.
- The person may feel that the type of service you are providing does not meet their needs.
- The person may not be able to meet with you during your working hours due to other commitments.

You may hear service users referred to as 'difficult to engage'. This label is often about blaming the service user for their reluctance to fit in to the service we are offering. However, as you can see from the list above, there are many reasons why a person may not wish to be involved with mental health services. Therefore, the skill of engagement is extremely relevant to mental health practitioners. In order to facilitate the process of engagement, the following tips could be useful.

Tips for facilitating engagement

- Wherever possible, we should aim to meet the person on their terms and in an environment that they are comfortable with. By offering a flexible and imaginative approach, an atmosphere of cooperation is more likely to be fostered from the outset.
- Be aware of the impact of the environment you are meeting the person within and attempt to make them comfortable in their surroundings. If it is on an in-patient ward, they may feel threatened and frightened, particularly if they are unsure why they are there, what might happen to them and whether they can leave.
- Adopt a friendly approach, using good eye contact and attentive listening skills which will help the person to develop trust in you.
- Offer a clear introduction of yourself which identifies who you are and why you are there.
- Allow the person to connect to you as a person as well as a mental health nurse.
- If the person is initially reluctant to engage with you, be persistent without being intrusive. Initial rejection could be part of the person's emotional problems and should not be viewed as the end of your attempts to initiate a relationship.
- Show you are willing and interested in getting to know the whole person and do not base your judgements of their needs solely on previous history or the opinion of other professionals who have been involved in their care.
- Respect the person's views and rights and work with them to define their needs and priorities. This may involve support initially with practical tasks which will enable the service user to view you as

useful to them. This can then provide the basis of the relationship and allow you to address more complex issues.

Maintaining therapeutic relationships

Maintaining therapeutic relationships is required to enable the delivery and review of a plan of care. Once the therapeutic relationship has been established, we should not assume that it is indestructible. There are a number of situations in which you may feel elements of your role as a nurse places the therapeutic relationship under threat.

The following scenarios are examples of these situations. Read the scenario and identify how you may respond to the situation in order to promote continued engagement. Suggested solutions are provided at the end of the chapter for each; however, these are not definitive and you may well have identified alternative approaches which are equally valid.

Scenario 1

Mohammed is a service user who you have been working with since the beginning of your placement. He has been involved with mental health services for many years and has been admitted to hospital under a Section in the past. Mohammed is very suspicious of mental health practitioners as he believes they have been involved in forcing him to take medication which has made him feel unwell. You have worked with him to understand his beliefs about medication and reconsider his perception of mental health practitioners.

Over the next few months Mohammed experiences a number of stressors in his life which have a negative effect on his mental health. He becomes withdrawn and is reluctant to see you. You share your concerns with your mentor and visit his home together. When you visit you see that his door has been boarded up from the inside and there are pieces of furniture in the garden which appear to have been thrown out of the window. You speak with your mentor who advises that a Mental Health Act assessment is required which will involve calling the police to break down his door. You are concerned that this will reinforce Mohammed's previous beliefs about mental health practitioners and destroy the relationship you and your mentor have developed with him.

Scenario 2

Jamal is a young man who has experienced psychosis for the first time. He is fully engaged in a package of care which involves a number of activities and groups aimed at supporting him to return to work and prevent future relapse. You are preparing to discharge him from mental health services, however his parents are very reluctant to agree to this decision. Anna is concerned that without the care package in place, Jamal will relapse and will end up back in hospital. Jamal's parents put in a complaint about you to the service team leader stating that you are not working for Jamal's best interests and they no longer want you to be involved in his care. You feel that if you withdrew, this would be detrimental to Jamal's progress due to the strength of the therapeutic relationship you have built with him. However, you are aware that Jamal is concerned about his parents' opinion and is highly influenced by their views.

Scenario 3

You have been working with Anna, a 45-year-old lady, who has a diagnosis of borderline personality disorder. Anna regularly expresses her wish to die and has taken overdoses in the past. When Anna is distressed, she contacts the team and demands that someone comes and sees her at that moment. You answer the phone to Anna and when you inform her that you are unable

to meet her demands, she tells you that if you do not come she will take an overdose. You are aware that this pattern of behaviour is a result of her need for support and her difficulties with asking for help in other ways. However, your mentor informs you that it is not helpful to respond to her threats as this reinforces this behaviour. You visit Anna the next day with your mentor as previously planned. She lets you in but tells you that you are just the same as the rest because you won't be there when she needs you.

Scenario 4

You are working on a busy acute admissions ward. Aaliyah approaches you to talk about her benefits which have recently been stopped due to her admission to hospital. You don't have time to talk with her about this and tell her that you will come over as soon as you get a minute. Aaliyah slams the office door and shouts 'I will believe that when I see it!'. You are aware that this issue is important to Aaliyah but you have been set a number of tasks by your mentor which you need to complete by the end of your shift.

Ending therapeutic relationships

The ending of a therapeutic relationship may occur for various reasons. Most commonly, as a student nurse, you will have completed your allocated time in the specific placement area and so will be moving on. It is important to consider how this is managed, as how relationships end can have significant implications for the service user. This is particularly relevant if the person has had a history of disruptive relationships in the past and therefore may perceive the ending of a relationship as a repeated rejection by someone they have grown to trust.

The parameters of the relationship, such as its nature, aims and duration, should be incorporated into the care plan. This can be discussed openly and mutually negotiated with the service user. There may be a natural ending to a therapeutic relationship when a goal within the care plan has been achieved. If this is not the case, you can use the following strategies to ensure that the ending of the relationship maintains its therapeutic focus.

Tips for ending relationships

- Be clear at the onset of the duration of your involvement with the service user.
- Remind them at regular intervals how much longer you will be working with them.
- Work with the mental health practitioner who will be picking up from where you left off. This may involve referring to another service, facilitating their introduction to the person over a couple of meetings or providing a detailed handover of what you have achieved.
- Plan for your final contact with the person. Ensure that this is focused upon evaluation and review rather than opening up new areas. This may involve a more informal interaction where you plan to do something that the person will enjoy.
- Indentify with the person what you have learnt from working with them and thank them for the opportunity they have given you.

🕭 Activity

1. Discuss the issue of ending therapeutic relationships with your mentor. Ask them to suggest ways in which you might approach this with the service users you will be working with on this placement.
2. Plan and implement this with a service user and reflect with your mentor on how they responded.
3. Identify what you can learn from putting this into practice.

Professional boundaries should be maintained throughout a relationship. This is stated within the Nursing and Midwifery Council Code (2008) and is therefore an ethical and professional responsibility. Part of establishing professional boundaries is about being clear about the purpose of the relationship, what it is and what it isn't. This contributes to ensuring the relationship does not foster a level of dependency that cannot be maintained. If you suspect that the service user is solely relying upon you to provide practical or emotional support, this may indicate that the relationship has developed to a level of dependency which is beyond professional boundaries. In order to address this, it should be identified at the onset that the relationship is not a friendship or permanent. Bearing this in mind, it is not appropriate to continue to maintain contact with a service user once your placement is complete.

References

Aldridge, J., 2006. The therapeutic relationship. In: Jukes, M., Aldridge, J. (Eds.), Person-centred practices: a therapeutic perspective. Quay Books, Wiltshire.

Barker, P., Buchanan-Barker, P., 2005. The Tidal Model: a guide for mental health professionals. Brunner-Routledge, London and New York.

Nursing and Midwifery Council, 2008. The code: standards of conduct, performance and ethics for nurses and midwives. NMC, London.

Rodgers, C., 1951. Client centred therapy – its current practices, implications and theory. Houghton, Miffin, Boston.

Further reading

Hewitt, J., Coffey, M., Rooney, G., 2009. Forming, sustaining and ending therapeutic interactions. In:

Callaghan, P., Playle, J., Cooper, L. (Eds.), Mental health nursing skills. Oxford University Press, Oxford.

Website

Centre for Mental Health: http://www .centreformentalhealth.org uk/

Possible solutions to scenarios

Scenario 1

You agree with your mentor that a Mental Health Act assessment is required in order to ensure Mohammed's safety.

1. Prior to the incident, you or your mentor could have worked with Mohammed to develop a relapse prevention plan or an advanced directive such as the ones described in Chapter 13. This would enable you and Mohammed to establish an agreement about how situations like this might be dealt with and what would make them less distressing for him. This would enable you to ensure Mohammed is in agreement with your actions and allow you to revisit this with Mohammed once he has recovered from the distressing event.

2. If this agreement had not been established, you could ensure that the way in which the Mental Health Act assessment was carried out was as sensitive as possible, based on what you have learnt about Mohammed and what helps him when he is distressed. You could then communicate this to the individuals involved in the assessment so they are clear how to respond to him and manage the situation in a way that is responsive to Mohammed's personal triggers and coping strategies. If Mohammed requires medication, you would also be able to explain to the care team his beliefs about different medications and what his preference would be.

3. Following the incident, it is important to explain to Mohammed why you took the actions that you did. Often people understand that this is in their best interests if the rationale is explained to them thoroughly. It may take some time for Mohammed to see your view and it is important to acknowledge the impact the event may have had on his perception of you and your mentor.

Scenario 2

You are clear that it is important for you to re-establish a relationship with Jamal's family in order to support his recovery and facilitate the maintenance of his natural social networks.

1. You may wish to start by establishing Jamal's views on his parents' concerns and how they are impacting on his perception of his own ability to move on from the service. This will determine the nature of the action you will take.

2. If Jamal is unsure about moving on against his parent's wishes, you may wish to initiate a series of group discussions involving Jamal and his parents. (The format and process of how this might work is described in Chapter 13.) This will enable you to work with the family as a whole to address their concerns and share information about the potential for recovery from mental health services. It will also enable you to acknowledge the family's anxieties and ensure that they are aware of your intentions.

3. If Jamal is happy with the prospect of moving on from services, you can support him to think about how he can express his views to his parents. This may involve considering the best way to frame his views and role playing the scenario in order for him to practise his responses.

Scenario 3

You acknowledge that you understand Anna's distress and frustrations with getting the help that she feels she needs. You explain that you are committed to her and her care but that you cannot respond to her in the way she expects due to the nature of your role and responsibilities to other people. You and your mentor suggest the following options and agree with Anna which she feels most comfortable with.

1. You set a time each day for Anna to talk to a member of the team for 15 minutes in addition to your fortnightly visits. If Anna is feeling distressed then she will use these phone calls to identify how she will manage her distress and consider personal coping strategies.

2. If Anna feels that she cannot manage her own distress and does take an overdose, she agrees to arrange an ambulance to A&E to receive medical intervention. Your mentor agrees with the A&E staff that they will inform you if this occurs.

3. You work with Anna to engage with a specific personality disorder service that provides you both with advice and direction on how to change unhelpful patterns of behaviour.

Scenario 4

You recognise that Aaliyah has been let down in the past by members of staff and you are keen to ensure that she does not feel that you are not interested in her concerns.

1. You leave your current task to speak with Aaliyah and identify a time when you will be able to speak with her about her concerns.

2. You consider the tasks you have been given to complete by your mentor and prioritise or delegate to other members of the team in order for you to find time for Aaliyah.

3. In your meeting with Aaliyah, you explain the challenges of meeting everyone's needs on the ward and explain that this is an issue that has no reflection on your commitment to her or her care.

8

Collaborative approach to nursing: assessment and care planning

CHAPTER AIMS

- To outline the different types of assessment and consider what is required for an effective holistic assessment
- To identify the advantages and disadvantages of the different resources that may be used to conduct an assessment
- To understand goal setting and a collaborative approach to care planning

Introduction

This chapter provides an overview of assessment and care planning in mental health nursing practice and examines ways in which you can develop your skills in this area during your practice placements. It introduces the concept of holistic assessment, considering some of the areas that this might cover. The section highlights the different types of assessment that may be used, resources for the collection of, and some examples of, questions you may want to ask. The chapter also reflects on the issues faced by mental health professionals when asking questions that they may find embarrassing or difficult. Risk assessment and management are addressed separately in Chapter 9.

Assessment provides the opportunity to develop an understanding of the person and to identify their needs, problems, strengths and goals. Following on from this it is essential to work with the individual and (where they are involved) their family in order to meet their needs, help them work towards dealing with their problems and realising their goals. This involves making sense of the information gained during assessment and using this to collaboratively develop a plan which will support this to happen. The last section will outline the process of planning care. It will also locate this in the context of the Care Programme Approach which provides the overarching framework for structuring assessment and care delivery in the UK.

Assessment

Assessment is an essential process within mental health nursing care. Participating in assessment enables the healthcare professional and the person in distress to identify and prioritise problems, strengths, needs and goals. It underpins the delivery of care and facilitates the decision-making process. As such, assessment forms an integral part of the nursing process (assessment, planning, intervention, evaluation). As Barker (2004) highlights, this involves aiming to gain an understanding of that person and their circumstances. In this respect, assessment should be a holistic process. This term is often used within nursing practice, however one of the criticisms levelled towards health care is that we don't always work with people holistically. In particular, mental health services have been criticised for tending to focus on problems alone without recognising people's strengths or the context in which they are managing their experiences. A holistic assessment will therefore explore and evaluate the resources an individual has, or has access to, and their environment. Who we are, the meaning and impact of any health-related problem may in part be influenced by our culture, sexuality and spirituality. Working with the 'whole' person therefore entails recognising and considering this.

 Activity

In the early part of your placement, identify the assessment frameworks or tools that are used in your practice area. This may involve:

■ Talking to your mentor about what frameworks or tools they use.

■ Looking at blank assessment forms.

■ Accessing individuals' multidisciplinary records (though it is important to bear in mind this may inform your perception of that person if you haven't already met them).

Review these frameworks in light of the list below. Do these attempt to collate holistic information? If not, what

information are they attempting to gain? What areas are being assessed? You might also want to think about whether these link with any of the theories covered in Section 1.

This will help you gain some familiarity with the aims of some specific types of assessment and with their structure, which will be useful when you conduct assessments in your own practice.

Areas that may be covered within nursing assessment include the following:
• Social networks and relationships.
• Description of the problems that the person is experiencing and the impact they are having (this may be symptoms of mental distress but may also include, for example, housing, relationship or employment difficulties).
• Family relationships.
• Past history such as health problems (physical and psychological), life events.
• Risk – current and/or past.
• Strengths, e.g. previous successes and areas of interest or enjoyment.
• Ways the individual uses to cope with their experiences (coping strategies).
• Medication – history, current, concordance and side effects.
• Housing and environment.
• Spirituality – spiritual beliefs and expression.
• Cultural beliefs and expression.
• Sexuality (or sexual health) – may include expression and impact of health problems and medication.
• Physiology, such as physical health, blood pressure, body mass index and physical expression of distress such as hyperventilation.
• Thoughts and emotions, e.g. thoughts about suicide or problems with mood.
• Non-verbal communication.
• Speech and expression.

- The individual's perception and meaning of their distressing experiences.
- Cognition – might include memory and orientation.
- Use of alcohol and illicit substances.
- Previous experiences of trauma and abuse.
- Occupation.
- Financial.
- Past treatment and support.

This is not a complete list but, as you can see, conducting a holistic assessment is extensive. It is important to consider this broad range of areas as this contributes to an understanding of that person and their context. It is also likely to facilitate a better informed, more accurate and therefore more effective process of making decisions, planning and delivering care. It also enables the health professional and person using the service to gain a picture of what is considered as 'normal' for that person in their life – a standard which is likely to differ for all of us. However, there are some challenges of examining assessment as a holistic process.

Gaining an understanding of people's experiences in their context (through holistic assessment) is important at whatever stage people come into contact with mental heath services and to recognise that circumstances will change. However, this may be more the focus of assessment when people are new to services, to that particular practice area or at a point before a change, such as discharge from a service or annual review.

According to the *Oxford English Dictionary* (Thompson 1996), to assess means to 'estimate the size or quality of'. Assessment in health care is clearly an essential process to help identify what support people would most benefit from. However, it is essential to bear in mind that its very purpose is to make judgements and that conducting an assessment involves exploring areas of a

> ### (♦) Reflection point
>
> Have a think about going to visit your GP for the first time, the first time you met your lecturer at university or when a new neighbour moved in next door.
>
> 1. How would you feel if these people were to ask you a question about each of the areas of your life identified above?
> 2. What would be informing how you responded to these questions?
>
> This reflection may be useful to keep and revisit when you have observed and/or participated in an initial assessment. At this point, it may be useful to consider the following issues to help you develop a reflective practice.
>
> 1. What are your perceptions of what a person may feel during an assessment?
> 2. What might inform how they respond to questions?

person's world that may be quite private and that they may not have shared before. This process will be informed by the rapport that is developed with service users and the values and beliefs of the practitioner and their organisation. It is a clinical skill which must be developed and used with sensitivity.

Assessment is a dynamic and ongoing process. In this respect the aim and purpose of assessment may differ depending on what context and setting you are working with someone in. For example, assessment plays a vital role in the following:

- Finding out whether someone who comes to A&E having taken a paracetamol overdose is likely to repeat this and needs ongoing support or used it as an impulsive way of coping with a change in their life.

- Finding out in what situations someone's derogatory voices are triggered and the way that they deal with this.
- Identifying what impact the side effects of newly prescribed medication are having.

This highlights that it is really important to differentiate between assessment and admission or acceptance by a mental health team. During an admission or being taken onto a community nurse's case load, it will be essential to conduct an assessment. However, assessment is a continual process that happens in many different settings. Identifying the different types of assessment and how this is conducted by nurses in your practice area would highlight this and help you plan for how to contribute to mental health nursing assessments. This might be something you want to discuss with your mentor or a practitioner in a question and answer session to find out more about how assessment is conducted in your practice setting.

Types of assessment

Assessment is a process which will draw on all your senses as well as the therapeutic skills that a nurse develops. Effective and sensitive communication alongside being alert to non-verbal and environmental cues is important for all assessments. However, methods of conducting an assessment could be divided into three main groups:

1. Observation.
2. Interviews.
3. Structured questionnaires.

Observation

This mode of conducting an assessment will entail gathering information that is observable. It can be informal such as taking into account the environment or a person's appearance (Ryrie & Norman 2009). How

people act, communicate and express themselves can also be observed. In this respect, observation often informs assessments of behaviour. Physiological basic observations may also be considered under this type of assessment as they provide access to information about measurable changes in physiology such as blood pressure and blood glucose. Different levels of structured observations may be common within a range of in-patient settings such as acute care, forensic and child and adolescent. These are often used as tools or interventions to help manage risk. However, these can also operate to inform nursing assessment as during these periods staff will be observing, in particular, behaviour and communication. This can also help inform the assessment of risk.

 Activity

The use of observation by looking at cues as to how individuals may present themselves, express themselves or their own environment is an assessment skill that you will be able to use in your placements throughout your training, if you are in the community, after you have been on a visit or if you are in an in-patient unit after spending one-to-one time with an individual. Consider the following:

1. What did you notice about the individual's body language and non-verbal communication (Sect. 1 and Ch. 7)?
2. What did you notice about the person's environment?
3. What might these have suggested about how they were feeling?

You may want to check these observations out with the nurse who you went on the visit with, a member of staff on the unit or the person's notes in order to get an insight into the 'norms' for that person and check out the accuracy of your observations. This could be something you document and communicate to other staff (all these processes could contribute to the achievement of your outcomes). It is also important to remember that our own norms and standards for environment may be different to what is a norm for another person.

Interviews

Interviews will involve gaining information from the individual and potentially others associated with their care through careful questioning and conversation. This tends to be a more formalised form of assessment where a professional will sit down with someone who uses services, skilfully ask questions and respond therapeutically to gain a picture of their current and past experiences. Clearly this is dependent on using interpersonal skills effectively and learning to really listen, so incorporates all those skills and approaches outlined in Chapters 3 and 7. Barker (2004) defines three different forms of interview and their role in assessment.

Descriptive

This includes gathering information to capture a broad overview of the person. It may also be helpful at initially establishing rapport and developing the therapeutic relationship. Open questions and statements alongside reflecting meaning back to people may be particularly helpful in this type of interview

Investigation

This relates to examining a specific area or problem in more depth. It may include considering connections between

thoughts, feelings and actions. Additionally, gaining some estimate of scale can be helpful when exploring an issue in detail. This may include the impact it has on that individual's life or their perception of its severity. Questions which incorporate scaling, clarifying statements and closed questions can also be helpful communication skills to use here.

Ongoing

Barker (2004) describes the therapeutic value in regular and ongoing meetings. In terms of assessment, these can help to clarify difficulties, consider solutions, establish goals and review progress. Using solution- and strengths-focused questions (see following sections) and clarifying meanings can be useful in this area.

While it is helpful to think about the different types of interview situation and how these may be used, it is important to note that an interview may change between these different types and there is overlap between each.

Structured questionnaires

There is a broad and extensive range of structured assessment tools. These instruments use specific structured questions or rating scales to attempt to provide quantifiable information on an individual's experiences. In this respect they often result in a numerical value or judgement according to a specific level (e.g. high, medium or low). Questionnaires may ask people to respond in a yes/no fashion or determine frequency or intensity by asking for a rating in response to a series of statements. These tools are often thoroughly researched prior to publication and being made available for use in clinical practice. This means that the tools have been tested to see whether they measure what they are supposed to (validity) and are consistent in doing this (reliability).

This type of assessment may also include tools used to examine a specific area such as a voice or activity diary.

Gamble and Brennan (2006) highlight that tools should be considered for how user-friendly they are, whether they are relevant to practice and easy to follow. This is important to remember, particularly as it is advised that some assessment tools require specific training. Training helps to ensure that the tool is used in the way it was intended and therefore that the reliability and validity are maintained. Additionally, some of the structured questionnaires can be quite technical or invasive in the questions that they ask and, therefore, using them requires this to be thought through and explored. Examples of questionnaire assessment tools include the following:

- Mini-mental State Examination – measurement of cognition and memory used in people with dementia.
- Liverpool University Neuroleptic Side Effect Rating Scale (LUNSERS) – used to measure side effects of antipsychotic medication.
- Becks Depression Inventory – used to rate low mood.
- Beliefs About Voices Questionnaire – examination of voice-hearing experiences and the individuals' perceptions of their voices.

Deciding on a type of assessment

Each approach to assessment has its strengths and limitations. As a practitioner you will be involved in using different types of assessment on different occasions. For instance, on an initial meeting with a service user, it may be most helpful to conduct an assessment via an interview to find out more about that person's difficulties, strengths and sources of support at the current time. This might indicate that experiencing anxiety is making it difficult for them to go out. At a further meeting, using a structured assessment tool can give you more information about the triggers and severity of their anxiety. If someone is acutely distressed and it is difficult for you both to find a common ground of verbal communication, assessment using observation may be most valuable. Gamble and Brennan (2006) warn of the dangers of using only one type of assessment as it is unlikely to be able to fully address the wide-ranging needs, wishes and strengths that an individual will have.

Each type of assessment has its advantages and disadvantages. For example, an interview assessment enables the service user to set the agenda and take more control within the assessment situation, yet it is a

---

⟲ Activity

Following on from the activity at the start of this chapter, identify what types of questionnaire tools are used in your practice area.

1. What are they designed to measure?
2. What is needed for their use, such as permissions, level of training?
3. When might they be used? This might be a stage in a person's care or in response to the identification of specific problems through other types of assessment.
4. What are the recommendations, if any, of how to respond to the results?

It may be helpful to talk to the staff in your placement area to answer these questions. As highlighted above, a number of the tools have also been researched so accessing published articles will also aid this.

subjective process which may be influenced by the values and beliefs of the practitioner and therefore is harder to measure change over time. Structured assessments offer more consistent measures in this respect but may be limited in what information they provide about the context of individual's experiences. Additionally, Chapman and Chessum (2009) highlight that the language that is used in structured assessments may not be meaningful to all cultures.

Preparing for assessment

Assessment is an ongoing process which is a core part of mental health practice across a diverse range of settings. Engaging in an assessment can be the first time that an individual has had contact with mental health services and a mental health professional (Chapman & Chessum 2009). In this respect the assessment process could play a significant role in forming their future perceptions of that service. This highlights the importance of a sensitive and understanding approach. In order to aid this, it is helpful to think about some key areas which should be considered prior to conducting any assessment.

Where?
- Where will the assessment be conducted?
- Is this space confidential and private?
- Have potential interruptions been planned for and minimised?
- Is the room as comfortable as possible?
- How are the chairs positioned to facilitate communication?
- Are there any safety issues that need to be addressed (such as lone worker policy or positioning within the home environment)?

When?
- When is the best time to conduct the assessment?
- What time of day may be preferred by the individual?

- Is there a time of day when this may be more easily facilitated, e.g. when an individual may be more able to concentrate, more likely to be awake?

Who?
- Who needs to be involved in the assessment?
- Has consideration been given to gender, culture or personal preference?
- Does the person require any support or is there anyone they would like involved such as an advocate, peer support worker?
- Is there any indication that the assessment should be conducted by a certain discipline or whether it should be a joint assessment between services?
- Are there significant others involved as carers – is there a need for a carers' assessment?
- Has the person given consent for a student to be involved?

How?
- What is the most appropriate method of assessment for this person and service?
- How are you going to approach the assessment? What will inform this?
- What issues of confidentiality need to be considered? How will this be communicated to the individual and the multidisciplinary team?
- How will the assessment be recorded?

Why?
- What is the purpose of the assessment?
- What information needs to be and should be examined?
- What will be done with this assessment information?
- What will it be judged against? How will this be evaluated?

This has provided an indication of some key areas that should be considered when conducting an assessment. It is proposed that asking these questions of yourself (and mentor) when involved in the assessment process will help enable the assessment to be as comfortable as possible for the person using services, but also ensure it is safe and effective.

It is important that you think about these issues when you are conducting assessments in placement settings. As this discussion has highlighted, you may be involved in using observation as an assessment skill. In conducting assessments, it is really helpful to observe different nurses conducting more formalised assessments (using questions or assessment tools) to reflect on the different approaches and skills that may be used effectively in assessment.

 Activity

After this opportunity, consider what skills the professionals used? What did the person with mental health problems respond to most in the assessment?

In conjunction with your mentor, develop an action plan for how you can get involved in conducting assessments in your placement area. Depending on the stage of your learning and placements, this may include the following:

- Contributing to a formal assessment by asking some questions in conjunction with a nurse.
- Contributing to the interpretation and documentation of an assessment.
- Leading an assessment with supervision/support from your mentor.
- Producing an action plan for developing assessment skills on future placements.

Sources of information

Conducting an assessment requires consideration of the sources of information that will be used in order to gain an

understanding of that person's experiences at that time. Most importantly this must begin with the person concerned. However, there are other important resources that can be helpful for the assessment. This will be both to gather data and make sense of this information. Table 8.1 outlines some examples of the other resources that a nurse might use in an assessment, and a brief overview of some of the issues that will need to be considered when using this information. You may want to add to the benefits and cautions outlined here.

Ideally, using a variety of resources assists in gaining a holistic view and will help inform any gaps in understanding that a person may not be able to share, such as when they were really unwell. There are challenges to this in terms of time, accessibility and resources. Nursing assessment has also been criticised for being too problem focused and requiring people to retell the same story (Watkins 2001), which highlights the importance of asking ourselves the questions of 'why' outlined above. This entails thinking about what information is needed and what might be the best source of information.

Assessment – some examples

The following part of this chapter provides some practical tools and information to help you start to get involved in the assessment process in your mental health placements.

This section examines using the interview approach to assessment. Here we highlight the different 'types' of question that can be used during interviews. Below are some examples of different forms of questioning style.

Open questions
- Tell me about how you have been feeling over the past couple of days?

Table 8.1 Sources of information for assessments

Source	Benefits	Cautions
Family members, significant others and carers	They may know the person best and sometimes be able to recognise changes that the person doesn't	Their family member is their priority and accessing support can be difficult. These issues might impact on how people perceive a situation
Past structured assessments	These can provide some information against which current ratings may be compared	If the assessments have been conducted by different people there can be different interpretations of the ratings and, therefore, the measure is more subjective than it appears
Past running records/notes	This can provide detailed information about a person's situation and, through analysis, some insight into what may help people cope or cause them stress	These do not always provide an accurate picture and inaccuracies can be constantly repeated if this is the only source of information that is used
Other professionals that may have been working with that person	This may help to provide additional insights into specific areas of need or strengths that a person may have had. It may also help to gain a broader perspective and, in some circumstances, some facilitators for building a relationship	Interpretations may be subjective and informed by that person's beliefs and values

- What have you found helps you when you start to feel anxious/down/the voices are bad?
- How have these problems impacted on your life?

Clarifying questions
- How often has this been happening?
- What time of day do you find the anxiety/voices/racing thoughts are at their worst?
- What time of day do you find the anxiety/voices/racing thoughts are at their best?

- Did you say that it was last July that your medication was changed?

Rating questions
- On a scale of 1 to 10, with 1 being the worst, how has your anxiety/voices/mood been today?
- On a scale of 1 to 10, with 1 being the worst, where would you like your anxiety/voices/mood to be next month?

- How effective has that way of dealing with your distress been for you? Would you say it has been high, medium or low?

Varying the types of questions used can take time and practice to build to using as a skilful approach. However, using open, closed and clarifying questions appropriately creates space for the person to share their thoughts, feelings and emotions but ensures you have an opportunity to clarify your understanding and interpretation of this. Rating questions can be really useful when people may struggle to verbalise some of these thoughts and feelings as well as providing an opportunity to start moving towards goal planning and setting. These rating questions are informed by a solution-focused brief therapy approach (see Ch. 6 for more details). Clearly conducting an assessment also involves using the other interpersonal skills that you have learned to respond to the individual.

Biographical narrative

This is an approach most commonly used in working with older adults. It focuses on the person's story and getting to know the whole person, moving beyond their identity as a 'patient'. This can be particularly important when working with people diagnosed with dementia and is influenced by Tom Kitwood's theories on 'personhood' and dementia (Kitwood 1997). He highlights the basic psychological needs of all human beings and that the individual's personality and biography will influence their experience of dementia.

Conducting a biographical narrative with a person within the context of a therapeutic relationship involves enabling them to tell their story. Therefore, during one-to-one sessions with the individual you would use open and unstructured prompts to help them tell their narrative and share what they perceive as important. For example, 'Tell me about your life, the things that stand out and are important to you'.

This might be something that you record in a written form with the person but may use more creative methods such as scrapbooks or photographs (this also shares some similarities with life story work). Photographs and memorabilia may be used as prompts for storytelling. Narrative in this respect can act as a therapeutic approach or intervention alongside providing a resource for assessment.

For example, Ray is on an assessment ward for older people. He wakes in the middle of the night at the same time every night and tries to get in to make a drink. He gets frustrated and verbally aggressive when the nurse guides him away from the kitchen. Through doing a biographical narrative with Ray, his key worker discovers that he was a night worker and that the time he wakes up reflects the break time during his shift.

This example highlights the potential impact of conducting a biographical narrative. Underpinned by the interpersonal skills examined in this book and with the support of your mentor, biographical narrative is an approach you might want to be involved in when in settings with older persons.

Asking the embarrassing questions

The chapter started by highlighting the importance of conducting a holistic assessment. Previously, services have been criticised for overlooking core parts of people's identity and experience within the assessment process, therefore failing to consider the impact of these on their lives. The areas that are often overlooked relate to people's spirituality, culture and sexuality (these are examples; there may be others). Some of the reasons that it may be difficult to explore these issues are that they are areas which may be more hidden, that we may not be used to sharing or talking about except with those whom we are very close to. It is also difficult to define what is meant by some of these terms.

Some of the ideas that people have when thinking about being 'a nurse' might involve thinking about the physical closeness and invasive techniques that this involves. However, as a mental health nurse, sometimes there are more implications for this in terms of the emotional and psychological closeness and invasiveness that this entails. We may be privy to the thoughts and feelings people have that they may not have shared with anyone, or only those very close to them. In this respect it is essential that these complex areas are handled with sensitivity in a way that respects the person's dignity. However, this also involves a recognition of the significance of these aspects of people's identity and the impact that mental health problems and using mental health services can have on these areas.

Outlined below are some suggestions for consideration in approaching topics or questions that may be perceived as sensitive by you or the person using the service.

Language

It is important to try and mirror the language that a person uses to describe a particular issue or experience. This not only demonstrates you are actively listening but also that you are respecting their values and beliefs in relation to the particular issue. There may be limits to this if derogatory language is being used.

Timing

This can be a difficult thing to judge and is often something that may be easier over time (though even experienced professionals may misjudge from time to time!). Clearly it also depends on the context in which you are engaged in the assessment as to how much flexibility there is on the time for asking more

sensitive questions. It is important to respond to the verbal and non-verbal cues from the person but it may be that some people feel they can be more open about these issues when they have had the opportunity to get to know you and build a rapport. This can mean it can be important to revisit these areas in later assessments. However, it also involves recognising that people make choices not to discuss these areas.

Your own views

Using some of the skills of self-awareness explored in Chapters 5 and 7, it is important to reflect on how you feel both about asking questions which may relate to sensitive topics and about those topics themselves. What are your beliefs in relation to these areas and what if any prejudices or stereotypes may you have? Reflecting on how you feel about asking questions about such issues is important and it's not uncommon to feel embarrassed, especially to begin with, to ask sensitive questions. In managing this feeling, it is important to use the sources of support and forums of reflection that you have available to you, such as supervision. There will also be times when it is appropriate to share this feeling, reflecting congruence within your personal interaction. Here is an example of how this may be phrased sensitively:

> *This question is sometimes awkward for people to answer and I find it a bit awkward to ask but it's an important part of getting to know you. I also want to make sure that you have the space and opportunity to share with me anything that you feel is important for me to know in relation to/for our continued work together.*

It also important to recognise that how we feel about a particular issue may inform some assumptions that can be made about how other people might feel, for instance being embarrassed to ask a question doesn't always mean that someone will find it embarrassing to answer and vice versa.

There may also be other questions or topic areas that you find difficult to ask about, particularly when first getting involved in the assessment process. These often relate to areas of 'risk' such as asking people about whether they have ever had thoughts about harming themselves or have ever made an attempt on their life. It is an important part of the risk assessment process to explore these areas and people can appreciate sharing these thoughts with someone who understands and doesn't judge them. Some of the suggestions offered above may also help you think through how to approach an assessment of these areas.

It is important that you talk these issues through with a mentor exploring what their perspective is on whether it would be appropriate for you to get involved in this in relation to the people you are working with on your placement.

Summary

In summary, therefore, for this part of the chapter we can consider the following:

- Conducting an assessment with a service user is a complex and important area. Its aim is to gain an understanding of that person in the context of their life and circumstances; to get to know the person and inform the nursing process of planning and delivering care.
- There are different types of assessment and a range of resources that may be used. The process has potential to be uncomfortable and invasive for the service user and must be approached sensitively in order to establish rapport and ensure the person's dignity is respected.
- It is also important to highlight that the line between assessments and delivering care is blurred. Through the assessment

process, the mental health nurse invests in establishing rapport and building the therapeutic relationship.
- Additionally, some approaches that may be used during an assessment can have therapeutic benefit themselves, such as the narrative approach or rating questions. However, it is essential that a focus is maintained on what happens to the information once an assessment is conducted and how to make sense of the information to plan and deliver care. This is the focus of the next section.

Planning for collaborative care

Care programme approach

In the advent of community care (see Ch. 1), the Care Programme Approach (CPA) was introduced by the Department of Health (DH; 1990) to promote a more integrated system to ensure that the different community services involved in a person's mental health care are coordinated and work together. The CPA framework outlines the requirements of health and social services to provide the following (Care Program Approach Association 2010):

- Assessment: to conduct systematic assessment of health and social care needs for people in secondary or specialist mental health services.
- Care plan: to develop a care plan which addresses these identified needs.
- Care coordinator: to identify a person responsible for keeping in touch with the individual, coordinate and monitor care.
- Review: to provide regular review and evaluation of care, changing the care plan as agreed.

Assessment, care planning, care coordination and review are therefore viewed as the 'cornerstones' of the CPA

(Care Programme Approach Association 2010). Over the past 20 years there have been a number of amendments at a policy level that have led to adaptations in the structure and language of the CPA process.

The CPA was modernised further by the Department of Health in 1999. This included increased emphasis on risk assessment and a requirement that the CPA include crisis and contingency plans. It also integrated the process of case management in the community with the CPA approach (DH 1999).

A partnership approach to the CPA is integral. The CPA has brought together systems within health and social care. As the CPA is one of the main frameworks for care delivery in adult mental health, a key part of the partnership approach is those that are built with service users and carers (DH 2006). However, the CPA has been criticised for failing to realise its aims in this area. It has been seen to be too problem focused and research has suggested many service users remain unaware of the existence of their CPA care plan (Rose 2003). These concerns prompted a review of the CPA and the introduction of new CPA policy in 2008 (DH 2008). *Refocusing the Care Programme Approach* (DH 2008) promotes a more service user-centred philosophy and

suggests the CPA has to be underpinned by recovery and social inclusion. This involves working towards strengths and goals alongside addressing needs and difficulties. It also highlights the need to help people maintain control over their own support.

Role of the care coordinator

A range of different mental health professionals can be care coordinators. Psychiatrists might be care coordinators to a large number of individuals but often manage this through seeing them as out-patients. If people have complex needs or need input in a number of different areas of their life, they may be referred to secondary mental health services and be allocated a care coordinator who is most commonly a mental health nurse or a social worker but who may also be an occupational therapist.

This key role involves developing and sustaining a therapeutic relationship with service users, liaising with other professionals and services, conducting assessments, delivering care and support but also coordinating the support delivered by others. Working in this way often involves adopting a case management approach (as highlighted by the amendments to the CPA policy in 1999). This is discussed in more detail in Chapter 15.

 Activity

Figure 8.1 is an example of a completed CPA care plan. Have a look at this care plan and think about what you notice. Are there any problems with it?

Have a look at the CPA care plan in Figure 8.2, completed about the same person in exactly the same set of circumstances. What differences do you notice from the first one? In particular, think about:

- documentation and record keeping
- delegation
- recovery
- language.

How does this compare to the CPA care plans you have seen on placement?

Continued

Field Social Services and Happy Meadows NHS Trust

CARE PROGRAM APPROACH CARE PLAN

Name: .... Joe Baines .... *D.O.B.* ...... 07/08/1977 ....

Healthcare No. ...H03/xxx./..4956...

NEW CARE PLAN:

Diagnosis: .... Schizo-affective ....
....

Summary of progress since last review: Joe deteriorated and suffered
a major relapse resulting in admission to acute services. He was non-
compliant with meds and services before admission.
....
....
....
....

Future care co-ordinator:................. Sarah Kingston ....

Future Medication: .... Risperidone 4 mg ....

Need identified	Action	Person responsible	Expected outcome
Lacks structured activity, gets bored during day	Refer to OT	OT, Pete Davis	Engagement in structured activity
Joseph was non-concordant with medication change on admission	Develop crisis contingency plan Review medication	CPN	Improved concordance with medication on admission
Problems with activities of daily living	Refer to OT and prompt during CPN visit for house clean	OT Pete, CPN Sarah	House kept clean and tidy
Problems with auditory hallucinations	Review medication	Dr Petal	Reduced symptoms

(A)

Fig 8.1 Completed CPA care plan

Continued

Field Social Services and Happy Meadows NHS Trust

CARE PROGRAM APPROACH CARE PLAN

Name: .... Joe Baines .... *D.O.B.* ...... 07/08/1977 ....

Healthcare No. ...H03/xxx./..4956

CRISIS CONTINGENCY PLAN

Key contact details should be provided of agreed providers of support.
Coping strategies and relapse signatures should be highlighted.

Early Warning Signs:

• Disturbed sleep

• Disrupting neighbours

• Acting bizarrely

Contact crisis team if early warning signs present

Next review date: ....

We agree to keep this care plan

Service User: ....   *Date:* ....

Consultant Psychiatrist: .... *Signed:* .... *Date:* ..19/09/2010..

Care co-ordinator: .... *Signed:* .... *Date:* ..19/09/2010..

given to:	**User**	☐	**Carer**	☐
	Consultant	✓	**Other**	☐
	G.P	✓		

(B)

Fig 8.1—cont'd

Field Social Services and Happy Meadows NHS Trust

CARE PROGRAM APPROACH CARE PLAN

Name: .... Joe Baines .... **D.O.B.** ...... 07/08/1977 ....

Healthcare No. ... H03/xxx./..4956

NEW CARE PLAN:

Diagnosis: .... Schizo-affective..disorder. ....

Summary of progress since last review: Joe had a short admission to the assessment unit last summer. This was precipitated by an increase in his negative voices following the breakdown of his long term relationship. Joe was involved in the recovery group whilst on the ward and feels this helped him to settle back into the house after he was discharged. Joe has re-established his relationship with his brother Jake following the letter he sent him. Joe visits Jake frequently and feels this really benefits him. Joe has taken up drawing again and feels that this sometimes helps him to block out the voices....

Future care co-ordinator:................ Sarah Kingston ....

Future Medication: .... Risperidone 4 mg ....

Need identified	Action	Person responsible	Expected outcome
Joe would like to work part-time and feels this would help him keep occupied during the day	To work with Joe to identify Joe's skills, interests and experience To organise a voluntary work placement for Joe to continue to build this experience	Pete Davis, Occupational therapist Kate Uniwin, Employment facilitator	Identified area of interest for employment Development of skills and experience to enable a supported employment opportunity
Joseph was worried about his medication being altered when he was admitted to hospital. He was also concerned about the safety of his house and this added to his stress	To work with Joe to develop an advanced agreement Joe would like this agreement shared with his GP, the crisis team and Jake	Joe Bains Sarah Kingston Dr Petal	Advanced statement agreed with the crisis team
Joseph finds it difficult to maintain his house, particularly when the voices are worse	For Joseph to be supported to use his **personal budget** to employ a cleaner	Joseph Baines Sarah Kingston	The recruitment and employment of a reputable company/individual to clean Joseph's house, one afternoon a week
	To complete a beliefs about voices questionnaire and use to inform work with Joseph on coping strategies To identify and provide information on local hearing voices network groups	Sarah Kingston	For Joseph and Sarah to have a more detailed understanding of the triggers for his negative voices and to develop a plan for support/dealing with these

Fig 8.2
Alternative completed CPA care plan

Planning care

A care plan provides an account of the work that the service users and the professionals supporting them will undertake to meet the individuals' needs and achieve their goals. It is described as the next stage in the caring process following assessment and diagnosis of problems and needs (Leach 2007). In this respect It should be based on an interpretation of the information gained during assessment. Well written care plans can aid continuity of care, facilitate interdisciplinary working and consistency between care providers. CPA provides one of the core frameworks for care planning and, in some services, this may be the only care plan that underpins care. However, in some areas where guidance is required on the short-term aims and direction of care (such as in-patient services), additional care plans will be developed.

The process of developing a care plan helps to (Callaghan 2006, Gega 2009):

- identify and clarify actions or interventions needed to reach a goal or address a problem
- develop and articulate a shared understanding between the nurse and the person on what needs/goals can be met and the priority of these
- set measures for how progress towards achieving these can be measured, therefore agreeing outcomes.

Care plans should be developed in collaboration with the service user and reflect their priorities and wishes (DH 1999, Rogers 2000). In this respect, care plans should be individualised. It makes sense that any plan of action is more likely to be successful if it reflects something that the individual would like to achieve. This level of ownership can help foster individual autonomy and taking on greater responsibility. However, there are times when this level of collaboration is challenging, in particular if an individual is severely distressed or the plan relates to an

issue defined as a problem by professionals or society rather than the individuals themselves, such as the management of certain risks. Rogers (2000) highlights that it is essential that these management plans do not replace collaboratively agreed care plans. Additionally, it is important that service users are given ongoing opportunities to be involved in planning their care if they are too distressed at certain times. There is also opportunity to be creative about how we access people's thoughts about their care and goals, such as for people who may find it difficult to verbalise their wishes at some points, providing them with the opportunity to write this down or express it in other ways. It may also involve changing language and amending the way in which problems are expressed (Gega 2009).

Before the care plan can be developed, the nurse and the service user need to agree the priority of needs and goals in order to plan. Having too many care plans can create confusion for the person and services, making ineffective use of resources and reducing the impact of the plan on patient care.

Care plans start with a statement which may be expressed as a problem, need or goal (Bauer & Hill 2000), such as:

> Joan states that she benefits from medication and is happy to take it. However, she is regularly forgetting to take her medication as prescribed, inhibiting its therapeutic effect. Joan needs to take her citalopram 20 mg every morning.
>
> Problem: Leon feels isolated and identifies this contributes to his low mood.
>
> Goal: For Leon to reduce his feelings of isolation by joining the lost ramblers group.

These statements may represent a plan to move towards a more long-term goal, for instance Leon's long-term goal might be to meet a partner or have a wider network of friends. It is important to highlight these plans as part of a long-term goal.

The statement of a problem or goal is followed by an outline of the objectives, which break this problem or goal down into more specific details. Objectives should be SMART: specific, measurable, achievable, realistic and time orientated. This is often best achieved by keeping things simple, having a plan that addresses one problem or goal:

> *Plan: For the next 7 days Joan will set her mobile phone alarm reminder every evening to alert her to take her citalopram the following morning.*
>
> *Plan: Joan's keyworker will provide Joan with a tick chart in order to record when she has taken her tablet (by next visit).*

This may be a useful prompt when writing, reviewing and evaluating care plans during your placements. It may be possible to contribute to the care plan process by, for instance, reviewing and evaluating a plan with a service user you are working with.

In this example the person responsible and the expected time has been included in the statement of objective, making it clear who is responsible and when the objective is expected to be achieved. It can take practise to develop objectives that are specific and measurable, particularly given that the nature of problems or the support required to reach goals may be complex.

Care plans therefore need to outline the action required to reach goals or address problems, resources that will be required, who is responsible for this, how and when progress towards this area will be monitored. This last point also highlights the importance of evaluating care plans. All plans should include the measurement of achievement within that plan and the date at which that measurement will be evaluated. This evaluation has to be documented within multidisciplinary team records and on the plan itself. It is also important that the essential requirements of

record keeping are attended to when documenting a care plan, including the person's name and healthcare number, the signature and discipline of the person writing the care plan and the signature of the person whose care plan it is.

The overview of the care planning process given here has provided an insight into how care plans may be structured and developed. It has outlined the importance of ensuring this is a collaborative process and that care plans are driven by the individuals' goals and the process of assessment. Transferring the care plan into action is the next part of the process and, for this to be successful, effective communication, negotiation, team-working and leadership skills may be required. Leading and managing care are explored in Chapter 14.

References

Barker, P., 2004. Assessment in psychiatric and mental health nursing. In search of the whole person, 2nd ed. Stanley Thornes, Cheltenham.

Bauer, B., Hill, S., 2000. Mental health nursing: an introductory text. WB Saunders, Philadelphia.

Callaghan, P., 2006. Essential mental health nursing skills. In: Callaghan, P., Waldrock, H. (Eds.), Oxford handbook of mental health nursing. Oxford University Press, Oxford.

Care Programme Approach Association, 2010. About the Care Programme Approach. Online. Available at:http://www.cpaa.org.uk/thecareprogrammeapproach (accessed June 2011).

Chapman, J., Chessum, C., 2009. Fundamental skills of mental health nursing. In: Clarke, V., Walsh, A. (Eds.), Fundamentals of mental health nursing. Oxford University Press, Oxford.

Department of Health, 1990. Caring for people. The Care Programme Approach for people with a mental illness referred to specialist mental health services. Joint Health/Social Services Circular. C(90)23/LASSL(90)11Department of Health, London.

Department of Health, 1999. Effective care coordination in mental health services: modernising the Care Programme Approach. HMSO, London.

Department of Health, 2006. Reviewing the Care Programme Approach 2006: a consultation document. HMSO, London.

Department of Health, 2008. Refocusing the Care Programme Approach; policy positive practice guidance. HMSO, London.

Gamble, C., Brennan, G., 2006. Working with serious mental illness: a manual for clinical practice, 2nd ed. Elsevier, Edinburgh.

Gega, L., 2009. Problems, goals and care planning. In: Norman, I., Ryrie, I. (Eds.), The The art and science of mental health nursing. A textbook of principles and practice. 2nd ed. Open University Press, London.

Kitwood, T., 1997. Dementia reconsidered: the person comes first. Open University Press, Maidenhead.

Leach, M., 2007. Planning: a necessary step in clinical care. Journal of Clinical Nursing 17, 1728–1734.

Rogers, P., 2000. Forensic nursing. In: Newell, R., Gournay, K. (Eds.), Mental health nursing: an evidence-based approach. Churchill Livingstone, Edinburgh.

Rose, D., 2003. Partnership, coordination of care and the place of user involvement. Journal of Mental Health 12 (1), 59–70.

Ryrie, I., Norman, I., 2009. Assessment. In: Norman, I., Ryrie, I. (Eds.), The art and science of mental health nursing. A textbook of principles and practice, 2nd ed. Open University Press, London.

Thompson, D. (Ed.), 1996. Oxford compact English dictionary. Oxford University Press, Oxford.

Watkins, P., 2001. Mental health nursing. The art of compassionate care. Butterworth Heinemenn, Edinburgh.

Further reading

Aston, L., Wakefield, J., McGowan, R., 2010. The student nurses' guide to decision making in practice. Open University Press, London.

Websites

The Care Programme Approach Association: http://cpaa.co.uk/thecareprogrammeapproach (accessed June 2011).

Department of Health: Effective care coordination in mental health services: modernising the Care Programme Approach – a policy booklet. http://www.dh.gov.uk/en/Publicationsandstatistics/Publications/PublicationsPolicyAndGuidance/DH_4009221 (accessed June 2011).

9 Working with people to make choices about their treatment

CHAPTER AIMS

- To recognise the differences between compliance and concordance approaches to making choices about treatment options
- To discuss the values and skills which aid and support concordance approaches in practice
- To identify the potential benefits of adopting a concordance approach to the management of medication
- To identify the challenges of implementing concordance approaches when applied to a mental health context

Introduction

Throughout this book we have written about approaches which encourage practice-based partnership and cooperation with the service user. The medical model has been criticised for contradicting this approach, due to the perception that decisions are often being made by medical practitioners about the best course of treatment based upon their professional expertise regardless of the service user's views. This approach is known as promoting 'compliance' and involves encouraging the person to adhere to a treatment regime which has been prescribed for them.

This chapter will discuss ways of working which support the service user to make choices about their treatment options based on knowledge and information given to them by the mental health practitioner. This is known as promoting 'concordance'. The principles of concordance approaches apply to making decisions about all treatment options, however this chapter will focus primarily on how it can aid the management of medication.

Compliance

Compliance in the context of health care is defined as 'The extent to which a person's behavior in terms of taking medications, following diets, or executing lifestyle changes, coincides with medical or health advice' (Haynes et al 1979).

In a mental health setting, people are sometimes reluctant to adhere to medical advice for a number of reasons:

- They may disagree that they have a mental health problem and therefore do not see the need to follow the advice or treatment plans devised by mental health professionals.

- They may experience negative side effects of prescribed treatments which they feel are more disabling than the problem itself.
- They may view the treatment prescribed as unhelpful and not appropriate to address the problem as they perceive it.
- They may want to maintain their current lifestyle or some elements of their mental health problems as it gives them pleasure or is a significant aspect of their identity.

⚙ Reflection point

1. Consider an aspect of your lifestyle which you enjoy, for example a hobby, social activity or a way of relaxing.
2. Reflect upon how you would feel if you were asked not to engage in this activity any more because you were told it is potentially damaging to your health or may impact negatively on your social functioning.
3. What would influence your decision whether or not to follow the advice?

A number of service users have expressed their dissatisfaction with this approach to practice. It has been identified as disempowering as it doesn't acknowledge the person's perspective or take into consideration their knowledge of themselves (Perkins & Repper 1996). Furthermore, if the person does not agree with the treatment, they are unlikely to follow the plan as prescribed and therefore medication may be thrown away or appointments missed which can be a waste of resources.

In some circumstances a person may have been viewed as unable to contribute to a decision regarding their treatment due to the seriousness of their mental health problem. In these situations it would be appropriate for a Mental Health Act assessment to be undertaken or an assessment of the personal mental capacity. Parts of this legislation allow professionals to administer treatment against the person's will if it is deemed in their best interests (see Ch. 4). However, it is important to acknowledge that if this is not the case, the person has the right to make an autonomous decision about their treatment even if the mental health professional feels that they could be putting their health at risk. See the scenarios below for examples.

1. John attends a drug and alcohol support service during the day and engages in the various therapeutic interventions which are aimed at reducing his drug use. However, in the evenings with his friends, he continues to smoke cannabis. The quantity and strength of the cannabis he smokes is seriously affecting both his physical and mental health, however it is how he keeps in contact with his friends and so he is reluctant to stop.

2. Sarah has been prescribed an antipsychotic which is known for causing weight gain. Despite the difficulties she is having with her voices, she is very conscious of her weight and feels her appearance is important to her self-esteem and wellbeing. She decides not to take her medication but will not discuss this with her care team because she is sure they will force her to go into hospital.

3. Wesley has been referred by his social worker to a group for young people who have experienced domestic violence. However, he doesn't want to talk about his feelings to a group of strangers. In order to avoid going to the group he has been missing appointments with his social worker and refusing to talk to his mum about how he is feeling. He is becoming extremely isolated, his mood is getting consistently worse and he is having thoughts of suicide.

In these examples it is evident that the service users are not complying with their treatment plan for a range of reasons which is having a detrimental effect on both their mental health and their engagement with mental health services. In these types of circumstances it is proposed a concordance approach would be more beneficial.

Concordance

Weiss and Britten (2003) state that 'concordance is fundamentally different from either compliance or adherence in two important areas: it focuses on the consultation process rather than on a specific patient behaviour, and it has an underlying ethos of a shared approach to decision making rather than paternalism ... it is not possible to have a non-concordant patient'.

If we break this statement down, there are a range of skills and values which are required if we are to promote concordance.

1. A willingness to work in partnership with the service user and acknowledge their values, perspective and expertise.

2. An awareness of how the service user may view you as a professional and how this may impact on their willingness to be open with you about their views of their treatment.

3. A purposeful effort to engage with the person and build a therapeutic relationship.

4. The use of communication skills which enable the person to be open with you about their perceptions of the treatment options available.

In addition to these core elements, there are areas of knowledge and various tools which can aid this approach. The first of these is knowledge of the treatment options available.

In relation to medication management, it is beyond the scope of this book to provide you with a detailed explanation of each of the medications used in mental health services and how they work. Box 9.1 contains a brief explanation of the groups of medications commonly used in mental health services.

Box 9.1 Medications commonly used in mental health services

Antipsychotics/neuroleptics

These drugs are used to treat psychosis which is characterised by the experience of unusual thoughts, perceptions and voices. People who experience these symptoms are often diagnosed with schizophrenia which is thought to be partly caused by an increase in communication between brain cells due to the overactivity of an excitatory chemical called dopamine. Antipsychotics bind to receptors in the brain to reduce the transmission of nerve signals and therefore make nerve cells less sensitive to dopamine. They can also cause disturbances to other chemicals in the brain which leads to side effects such as restlessness, parkinsonism, low blood pressure and erectile dysfunction. Long-term use can lead to permanent side effects such as tardive dyskinesia which is characterised by repeated jerky movements. Different antipsychotics can be tried in order to reduce side effects and the lowest possible dose should be administered. Newer antipsychotics claim to cause fewer side effects because they act more selectively on the dopamine receptors. These are known as atypical antipsychotics.

Continued

Box 9.1 Medications commonly used in mental health services—cont'd

Antidepressants

These drugs are used to treat moderate and severe depression which is thought to be partly caused by a reduced level of neurotransmitters in the brain which stimulate brain activity (e.g. serotonin). Antidepressants work by increasing the level of these excitatory neurotransmitters by blocking their reuptake or preventing them from being broken down. It takes 10 to 14 days for antidepressants to reach a therapeutic level, however temporary side effects can happen immediately. There are three main types of antidepressants: tricyclic (TCAs), selective serotonin reuptake inhibitors (SSRIs) and monoamine oxidase inhibitors (MAOIs). TCAs can be very dangerous in overdose and MAOIs react with certain foods such as cheese to cause high blood pressure and headaches. As a result of this, SSRIs and TCAs are most commonly prescribed.

Mood stabilisers

These drugs are given to people who experience extreme fluctuations in their mood and are often diagnosed with bipolar affective disorder (also known as manic depression). The medication reduces the intensity of the extreme moods and helps to reduce the frequency of mood fluctuations. Lithium is commonly prescribed as a mood stabiliser which requires careful blood level monitoring due to its potential to be toxic. It can lead to side effects such as nausea, drowsiness and weight gain. If the person experiences side effects such as blurred vision or a rash, the medication should be stopped. It may also affect the function of the kidney and thyroid, therefore these are also monitored. Other mood stabilisers are available if lithium therapy is unsuccessful or unsuitable for the person.

Anxiolytics/antianxiety

These drugs are used for short-term relief of severe anxiety. There are two types of drugs used to reduce anxiety: benzodiazepines and beta blockers. Benzodiazepines reduce the brain activity to induce a sedative effect which aids relaxation. Beta blockers reduce the physical symptoms of anxiety such as increased heart rate and palpitations by blocking receptors and stopping the effects of adrenaline on the body. Benzodiazepines can cause low motivation, slower reactions and dizziness. If they are withdrawn quickly, they can cause increased anxiety, restlessness and nightmares.

Hypnotics

These drugs are prescribed for people who are persistently having difficulty getting to sleep or staying asleep. They are recommended if alternative non-medication options have not been effective and lack of sleep is having a detrimental effect on health. They should be used as a short-term remedy to reestablish sleep patterns. They work by depressing the brain function by reducing communication between the nerve cells which slows brain activity. The type of sleep that is induced when taking hypnotics is

> **Box 9.1** Medications commonly used in mental health services—cont'd
>
> different to normal sleep and therefore people often describe feeling hungover the following morning. They can cause dependence and they become less effective over time which leads to people needing an increased dose. Withdrawal from hypnotics can also be very distressing as a result of possible increased anxiety, nightmares and hallucinations. A common hypnotic medication used in mental health service is zopiclone. Alternatively, benzodiazepines can be used.
>
> **Antidementia**
>
> These drugs are prescribed for people who have a diagnosis of Alzheimer's disease to improve the symptoms of dementia. They work by preventing the breakdown of a chemical in the brain called acetylcholine which increases the person's alertness and slows down deterioration in the brain associated with Alzheimer's disease. They do not prevent the long-term progression of dementia and there is a gradual loss in improvement after they have been stopped. Side effects can include difficulties with urinating, vomiting and diarrhoea.

We recommend that in order to develop your knowledge base in this area, you complete and repeat the following activity. We suggest that this will enable you to relate the information regarding medication to people you meet, which is a helpful way of remembering this material. It also contributes to your learning in achieving your Nursing and Midwifery Council (NMC) competencies and essential skills (NMC 2010). We have recommended some texts which may be helpful in this area at the end of the chapter.

Once you have developed your knowledge of the medication options, it is then important to consider how you will present this information to the service user in a way in which they can understand the potential benefits and limitations. This aims to enable the service user to make an informed choice about their medication and is known as an educational intervention. Below you can see an example of how you might describe an atypical antipsychotic.

 Activity

1. Consider a small number of service users you meet in practice on each placement.
2. Identify their diagnosis and the medications that they have been prescribed.
3. Use the *British National Formulary* (BNF), medication-focused texts, National Institute for Health and Clinical Excellence (NICE) guidelines and the person themselves to identify:
   - the type or classification of medication they have been prescribed
   - the dose and frequency that they take the medication
   - the side effects that they experience and how they manage them
   - their view of taking the medication and the impact it has on their mental health.

Example: describing an atypical antipsychotic

Nurse: Hi Jenny. Last time we met we said we would have a chat about the medication you have been taking. You said you are having some doubts about continuing to take it. Is that still OK with you?

Jenny: To be honest, I'm not sure I want to take anything. I've heard some really scary things about what these tablets can do to your mind and I would rather stick with my herbal stuff.

Nurse: OK, I would be interested to hear what you have heard about the medication and the herbal remedies you mentioned. But before you make a decision, shall I tell you a bit more about the medication and you can see what you think.

Jenny: Yeah, I don't suppose there is any harm in it.

Nurse: Well, the medication that Dr Petal has prescribed for you is an atypical antipsychotic. This means it is one of the newer types of antipsychotic medications which work in a different way to the older types. The theory is that the voices that you hear are partly caused by a chemical in your brain called dopamine. This is a type of neurotransmitter which has been found to influence thoughts, emotions, mood and perceptions. It carries messages across the nervous system and sends signals which tell your brain how to respond. Some people have too much of the chemical and some people are very sensitive to it and so the medication works by blocking the chemical or reducing the amount that is produced. This doesn't fix the problem but can reduce the symptoms you might experience like your voices.

Jenny: OK that makes sense.

Nurse: Perhaps we can draw a diagram together of how this might look.

Jenny: Yeah that might help.

Jenny: So why have I being feeling all sleepy? I'm finding it really hard to concentrate on reading a book or watching TV. I've heard other people say they have had the shakes and that they might never go away.

Nurse: This is because of the side effects of the medication. It can also disrupt how other chemicals in your brain work and everybody seems to respond differently. What Dr Petal has done is started you off on a small dose and he will gradually increase it until it makes a difference to your voices. At the same time we would be monitoring any side effects. If the side effects were causing you problems then we would try a different type of medication.

Jenny: OK, I will have a think about what you have said and let you know.

Nurse: That's fine, I will leave this information leaflet with you so you can have a read and we can talk through any questions you have next week.

Key features of the interaction

- Jenny has started taking the medication without a clear idea of how it works or how it might affect her. This was affecting her beliefs about her medication and her motivation to continue taking it.
- Jenny is considering stopping her medication but feels able to speak openly with the nurse about this. This illustrates the presence of a therapeutic relationship and allows the nurse to discuss Jenny's beliefs about her medication.
- Jenny has got some ideas about alternative treatment options. The nurse acknowledges this and is open to exploring her ambivalence and uncertainty about her treatment.

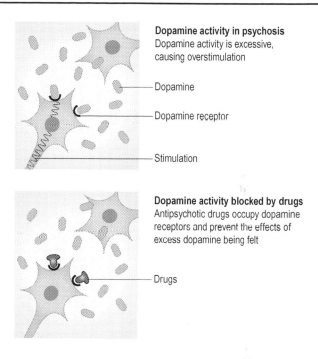

Fig 9.1 Action of antipsychotics

Dopamine activity in psychosis
Dopamine activity is excessive, causing overstimulation

— Dopamine

— Dopamine receptor

— Stimulation

Dopamine activity blocked by drugs
Antipsychotic drugs occupy dopamine receptors and prevent the effects of excess dopamine being felt

— Drugs

- Information about how the medication works is given in a clear and factual way.
- Different methods of presenting the information are used.
- Jenny is given the opportunity to ask questions and there is a focus on what is important to her
  (i.e. side effects, practical issues).
- Her perception about how the medication is affecting her is the central feature in the decision-making process illustrating a collaborative approach to decision making.
- The option to make changes based on her views of how her medication is affecting her is clearly given.
- The conversation is left open and plans are made to revisit it at the next session.

Other ways of promoting concordance are known as 'behavioural interventions' which aim to help service users think about how medication best fits with their daily routines. This might involve working with a person who finds it difficult to remember to take their medication. This may mean they are not getting a therapeutic dose or that they are taking extra to compensate when they have forgotten. Behavioural interventions would look at ways of reminding the service user and helping them to integrate taking medication into their daily routine. Alternatively the service user may be finding that the side effects of the medication are interfering with their day-to-day lives. In Jenny's case, a behavioural intervention might look like this:

Nurse: At our last session I remember you telling me your new medication was making you sleepy and affecting your concentration. How are you finding that now?

Jenny: It seems to have gotten worse now Dr Petal has increased the dose. The worst thing is I'm falling asleep during the day and then can't get to sleep at night. It's driving my boyfriend mad.

Nurse: Perhaps we can have a think about how we might improve this for you?

Jenny: Yeah that would be good. I have found my voices have got less intense but I'm not sure if that is just because I'm half asleep all the time.

Nurse: OK, do you have ideas?

Jenny: I'm not sure how much I'm allowed to mess around with it. At the moment I take the big dose in the morning and the smaller one at night. Is there any reason for that?

Nurse: Well you used to hear your voices louder around midday

Jenny: Yes but I haven't noticed that recently.

Nurse: Well, Dr Petal was thinking the larger dose might help with that but what were you thinking about the dose?

Jenny: Well I thought if I take the big one at night that might help me to sleep.

Nurse: Good idea, and the smaller dose in the day is less likely to affect your concentration.

Jenny: OK I will give it a go and let you know.

Nurse: That's fine. Will you also jot down how your voices are at different times of the day? That way we can see if the time you take your meds has any impact on how they work for you.

Jenny: Will do

Nurse: I will let Dr Petal know what we have decided to do and see if he has any ideas.

Key features of this interaction
- The nurse revisits the area that is important to Jenny and explores her current views.
- The nurse uses language which reinforces that this is a partnership process.
- The nurse answers Jenny's questions with a simple and accurate answer.
- The problem is approached collaboratively. Jenny is encouraged to think of solutions and an action plan is made on how to implement the solution.
- Plans are put in place to evaluate the success of the solution.

The final element of concordance is around making longer term plans with the service user about how their medication fits with future goals. For some people, alternative coping skills will be developed and they may wish to reduce their medication and eventually stop taking it. By using the skills identified above, this can be a highly positive process whereby the person feels in control of their mental health and supported in developing their independence from mental health services. For others, the continuation of medication may be helpful and it is important to consider with them how it will continue to be an assistance rather than a hindrance to them reaching their desired future.

References

Haynes, R.B., Taylor, D.W., Sackett, D.L., 1979. Compliance in health care. Johns Hopkins University Press, Baltimore.

Nursing and Midwifery Council, 2010. Standards for pre-registration nursing education. NMC, London.

Perkins, R., Repper, J., 1996. Working alongside people with long term mental health problems. Stanley Thornes, Cheltenham.

Weiss, M., Britten, N., 2003. What Is concordance? Pharmaceutical Journal 271, 493.

Bressington, D., Wilbourn, M., 2009. Medication management. In: Callaghan, P., Playle, J., Cooper, L. (Eds.), Mental health nursing skills. Oxford University Press, Oxford.

Healey, D., 2008. Psychiatric drugs explained. Elsevier, Edinburgh.

Further reading

British Medical Association and Royal Pharmaceutical Society, 2010. British national formulary. BMJ, London.

Websites

NICE guidance on medication adherence: http://www.nice.org.uk.

Mind: service user information and opinion on medications used in mental health: http://www.mind.org.uk.

10 Working with people who hear voices or express unusual beliefs

CHAPTER AIMS

- To describe a series of psychosocial interventions which will include:
  - responding to unusual beliefs
  - assessment of voices and unusual beliefs
  - coping skills enhancement
  - testing usual beliefs
  - motivational interviewing
  - working with families
  - relapse prevention
- To identify how they might be applied to your mental health nursing practice.

Introduction

This chapter will describe a number of interventions which may be helpful when working with people who hear voices or express unusual beliefs. These experiences are often termed hallucinations and delusions and are viewed as symptoms of psychosis. People who have these experiences may be given a diagnosis of schizophrenia or mania. The interventions described here can also be useful when working with people with a range of other mental health problems and will add to your tool box of possible approaches to consider when you are planning care.

The approaches are underpinned by the Stress Vulnerability Model which is described in Chapter 3 and often come under the umbrella term of psychosocial interventions. They attempt to enable service users to develop their personal and environmental protective factors, minimise the influence of vulnerabilities or reduce current stresses. This is with the overall aim of supporting the service user to develop self-management strategies and promote a sense of personal control over their mental health. It is important to recognise that these interventions are not the starting point for therapeutic work. They are sometimes seen as a quick practical solution to a person's problems. This approach overlooks the importance of engagement, assessment and developing a shared understanding with the service user (Mills 2006).

Before you begin to work with people who are experiencing psychosis it is essential to consider how their experiences might influence your approach. You may discover that the person finds it difficult to concentrate for long periods of time, keep appointments or complete tasks in between sessions. Some people do not feel motivated to take an active role in their care and are not used to being asked for their input and views. There is a possibility that a person's strange thoughts or voices might become prominent during a session, particularly if it is a new and potentially threatening situation. This will often mean a more flexible or creative approach is needed, which takes into consideration these possible obstacles and adjustments should be made in response.

Responding to people who express unusual beliefs

Students often describe knowing how to respond to people who express usual beliefs or strange thoughts extremely challenging. There are conflicting ideas about the best way to respond and it is likely that you will observe a number of different approaches in practice.

Case history

Client experiencing an unusual belief

You meet James at his home with your mentor. He tells you that the cracks in his wall are there to allow his neighbours to spy on him and report back to the government on his whereabouts and actions. James is extremely distressed by this and is asking you and your mentor to do something about it.

Possible responses that your mentor could give:

1. Your mentor tells James that the cracks are not there for his neighbours to spy on him and that his belief is a symptom of his mental illness. Therefore you and your mentor won't take any further action.
2. Your mentor doesn't mention the cracks in the wall but recognises that James is upset and offers him comfort and support with his distress.

She manages to distract James from his thoughts and he stops asking her to take action.
3. Your mentor talks with James about what makes him think that the cracks are there for his neighbours to spy on him, and explores the ideas which are underpinning his belief. They talk about this for some time and James seems to start to doubt his belief slightly. However, he would still prefer for you and your mentor to arrange for the cracks to be filled in. Your mentor tells James that she appreciates his view and concerns but sees the cracks in the wall as a normal occurrence and so doesn't feel that it is necessary to have them filled in.

Reflection point

- What do you think about these responses?
- What might be the implications of each of the responses above?

Response 1 could be underpinned by the practitioner's view that unusual beliefs should be challenged and failure to do so can result in the practitioner colluding with the service user and further confirming their belief. This approach can have a negative effect on the therapeutic relationship as the service user may not feel that you are making an effort to understand his distress. It also reinforces the idea that the practitioner is the expert and that their version of the truth is more valid than the service user's. This implies an unequal position and contradicts a collaborative approach to working.

In response 2 the mentor is adopting a more humanistic approach by focusing on the emotion arising from the belief rather than the belief itself. This can be helpful in the short term to alleviate the person's immediate distress and may strengthen the therapeutic relationship as the service user finds the mentor supportive and understanding. However, the distress is likely to return when the person refocuses on the belief as it has not been explored or addressed.

Response 3 is informed by a more collaborative approach. The mentor acknowledges the service user's belief and suspends her own judgement of its accuracy until they have had an in-depth conversation about it. This offers the mentor the opportunity to encourage the service user to look for evidence, which supports or conflicts with their belief, in an attempt to encourage the service user to question their belief, which may reduce their conviction in it. It also enables the exploration of the meaning of the belief to the person and how this is influenced by their previous life experiences. This process will often need repeating and it may take some time to have an impact. It is therefore appropriate to be honest with the service user about your perception of their belief. This communicates genuineness and allows the service user to see that while you are open to discussing their view, you do not agree with it and therefore are not confirming it in any way.

Response 3 is based upon the following assumptions about the most effective way of responding to a person's unusual beliefs, which is informed by the Stress Vulnerability Model (Zubin & Spring 1977):

- Unusual beliefs are best understood in the context of the person's past experiences, their current perceptions of themselves and their perception of the world around them.
- They are on a continuum with normal psychological functioning and are an extreme form of something that we all experience. For example, many people hold suspicious beliefs despite having no evidence to support them. These beliefs

influence their thoughts, actions or response to specific situations.
- The development of unusual beliefs can be a coping strategy which helps the person to deal with underpinning distressing experiences.
- The experience of unusual beliefs and the person's conviction in them can fluctuate and often increase during periods of stress (Gamble & Brennan 2000).

Assessment of voices and unusual beliefs

The in-depth assessment of unusual beliefs and voices is essential when considering the best way to help the person to cope with them. It can also help service users to make sense of their experiences and find their own meaning or explanation for them. There are a number of specific assessment tools which can guide you through this process, however they will commonly focus on the following areas:

For the assessment of voices:
- The characteristics of the voice, e.g. identity, gender, age.
- What the voice is saying.
- The person's explanation of how the voice is heard, e.g. telepathy, thought insertion from TV or radiowaves.
- What it means to the person to hear voices, e.g. they are gifted, having a spiritual experience or going mad.
- Whether the voice commands them to take a specific action and, if so, how easy they find it to resist the command.

For the assessment of unusual beliefs:
- The central theme of the belief, e.g. persecution, monitoring, fear of others.
- The rules and assumptions within the belief, e.g. everyone hates me, people are watching me, people are dangerous.
- The specific situations where the belief causes problems, e.g. going out in public,

speaking to people in shops, maintaining contact with family and friends.

- How much conviction the person has in the belief.
- How distressed they are by the belief.
- How much time they spend thinking about the belief.

General assessment of voices or unusual beliefs:

- How easy they are to ignore.
- What the triggers are.
- What makes them better or worse.
- How they cope with the problems that they cause.

(Adapted from Mills 2006)

Once a thorough assessment has been completed it is also important to check that you have a shared understanding of the service user's experience. This can be achieved by feeding back your ideas in small parts and explaining some of the connections you are making. At each point it is important to ask for the person's views on your interpretation, invite them to give their perspective and to identify points which they feel have been missed. This will allow for the picture to slowly build and ensure you have established a shared understanding of the person's experiences on which you can base further interventions.

Coping skills enhancement

When working with someone to develop their coping strategies, there are three areas which should be taken into account:

1. Coping strategies to enhance – these are ways of coping which the person already finds helpful but that they do not always use.
2. Coping strategies to reduce – these are ways of coping which the person already uses but that have harmful effects or lead to longer term distress.
3. Coping strategies to introduce – these are coping strategies which you and the

service user agree may be helpful to try out in light of what you have learnt about their current effective ways of coping.

The first step is to look at the person's current ways of coping. This reinforces the message that they already have resources which they have developed and focuses on their existing strengths. It can be helpful to ask the person to think of a recent time when they have felt distressed by their voices or beliefs and ask them to identify what they did, what they thought about and how it impacted on how they felt. This will allow you to recognise the style of coping that the person finds most helpful which can often be classified into:

- Behavioural – an action the person takes.
- Cognitive – a way of thinking.
- Sensory –the use of touch, taste, smell or sound.

Table 10.1 gives some examples of each.

Once you have identified these helpful coping strategies, you can suggest ways of increasing their effectiveness by encouraging the person to use them sooner and more frequently. You may also be able to suggest other ways of coping which may have the similar effect that the person is looking for. For example:

- Distraction – a way of thinking or behaving which removes focus on the voice/belief.
- Interaction with the voice – a way of responding to the voice which reduces its intensity.
- Testing out the belief – a way of looking for evidence to reduce conviction in the belief.
- Relaxation – a way of reducing the distress caused by the voice/belief.
- Accessing additional support – a pathway to a person or a group able to offer reassurance, a different perspective or a listening ear.

There may also be coping strategies, however, that the person finds helpful in the short term but that can have negative

Table 10.1 Examples of coping strategies

Behavioural	Cognitive	Sensory
Talking to others Exercise Completing tasks around the house Reading Playing an instrument Taking extra medication Talking to the voice or telling it to go away	Ignoring the thought/voice by thinking about something else Thinking about things which tell you the voice or belief is not true Repeating phrases in your head which you find soothing or reassuring	Aromatherapy Eating Listening to music Having a bath Relaxation/ breathing exercises

consequences in the longer term or lead to behaviour which is potentially harmful to the person's wellbeing. These would be coping strategies which you would be aiming to reduce. Consider the following case histories.

1. Ellen finds smoking cannabis enables her to relax and block out distressing thoughts. However, there is potential for this coping strategy to become uncontrolled leading to drug dependence, exacerbation of voices or thoughts, financial problems, reduced motivation and increased isolation.

2. Sean finds talking to his voices is the only way to quieten them. He usually does this in public by pretending to talk on his mobile phone. However, when he is at home, at times he becomes very angry with what they say and shouts and swears at them loudly. His neighbours have put a complaint in to the council about the noise and he has been given a formal warning.

3. Li believes that his ex work colleagues are involved in planning a terrorist attack in the city centre. He relieves his anxiety about this belief by phoning the police to report them. The police

assure him that they are investigating his suspicions and monitoring the situation, however Li continues to ring daily to receive updates. The police are becoming less tolerant and some refuse to take his call which causes him increased distress and worry.

4. Geeta hears a voice which she recognises as a girl who bullied her at school. The voice tells her to cut her arms and gets increasingly louder if she doesn't follow through with this command. She experiences immediate relief from the voice once she has cut herself but feels ashamed of the visible cuts and embarrassed when colleagues at work see them.

These ways of coping may be the only way the person is able to feel in control of their distress and therefore they may be reluctant to consider alternatives. It may take time for them to agree to work with you on trying out other ways and it will be important to provide high levels of support to enable the person to feel safe to do so. Quite often a less harmful version of the same coping method can be identified which will maximise the beneficial effects and reduce the potentially damaging ones.

Activity

For the examples given above, identify the following:

1. What is the effective part of the coping strategy that is being used and why?
   a. distraction
   b. relaxation
   c. interaction
   d. testing
   e. social contact.

2. An alternative coping strategy for Geeta in example 4 might be to flick an elastic band on her wrist or use an ice cube. This would enable her to respond to her voice without experiencing the shame and embarrassment she feels from how others respond to her cuts. What do think could be alternative coping strategies for examples 1, 2 and 3?

3. How would you encourage the people in these examples to consider these alternative coping strategies?

Testing unusual beliefs

People who experience unusual beliefs often have some common thinking styles which lead to a higher level of conviction in the belief and attempts to control the distressing emotions which arise from it by engaging in protective behaviours. Examples of these thinking styles include:

- Looking out for signs which confirm the belief and ignoring evidence which does not support it.
- Being preoccupied with the belief and continuously looking for evidence which confirms its truth.
- Misinterpreting coincidences or everyday experiences as evidence to support the belief.
- Jumping to conclusions quickly based on small amounts of evidence.

Stage 1

When encouraging the person to test the belief, it is important to take into consideration their thinking style and help them to recognise when it is influencing their thoughts and responses. This may involve starting with a belief that they have

had in the past which they have later realised was wrong, or identifying a time when they have jumped to the wrong conclusion. You may also wish to give an example of a belief that you have held in the past but have now revised in light of your experiences and the views of others. This starts the process off in a way which is non-threatening and reiterates the message that these thinking styles are common and something that we all experience to some degree.

Stage 2

The next stage of testing the belief is to encourage the person to identify the evidence they have which supports it and the evidence against it. You can then help them to assess the quality of this evidence by taking into account the potential misconceptions arising from the thinking styles you have already discussed. For example:

Nurse: What makes you think that the cracks in the wall are there for your neighbours to spy on you? (Identifying the evidence for.)

James: Well I've seen them look at me a certain way which tells me that they have been watching me. Anyway it's all over the news about CCTV and surveillance. This is just another way of the government keeping an eye on me.

Nurse: Are there any other reasons why there may be cracks in your wall? (Identifying the evidence against.)

James: Can't think of any, I suppose sometimes they just appear.

Nurse: We have talked about how it is easy to jump to conclusions, especially when we are feeling a little self-conscious or anxious. Do you think that you could be reading a little more into the way your neighbours are looking at you? (Recognising thinking styles.)

James: No way, they are definitely looking at me funny.

Nurse: That must be tough to see. Perhaps they are looking at you in a funny way, but that may be for different reasons to your idea about the cracks? (Validating the perception while introducing doubt.)

James: Maybe. I suppose I could be joining dots which don't really join. Like you did when you thought your friend wasn't speaking to you and she had just lost her mobile phone.

Nurse: That's right, it is easily done.

Stage 3
Now you have introduced doubt in the belief, you can support the person to look for further evidence to test its accuracy. This will involve working together to find a simple way of testing the belief which is safe for the person. The test should be thoroughly considered and take into account the person's predictions about the outcome of the test, any concerns they have about undertaking the test and how alternative outcomes to the ones they predict may influence their belief. In James's situation, the test might involve him going to his neighbour to ask to borrow some coffee. James may predict that the neighbour will respond to him in a negative way or refuse to lend him some coffee. If this is the case, it would confirm that there are some problems with their relationship which could be resolved. If not, it would add more doubt to James's conviction in the belief. Once the test has been carried out, time should be spent discussing the outcome and its meaning to the service user.

This approach can also be used to help a person gain control of their voices by testing the power the voice has over their actions or the validity of what the voice is saying to them. For example, if the voice is commanding them to carry out an action, what happens if they do not follow through with the action? Or if the voice is telling them they are insignificant and unlikeable, what evidence is there against this?

The key to this approach is to enable the person to lead the process in order to feel safe within it. It may involve the person changing a behaviour which they have used to protect themselves for many years or challenging thoughts which are an integral part of their belief system. This process may take time as change will require the person to place themselves in an uncomfortable position. It is important to consider with your mentor how you will contribute to this intervention and how it fits with the person's wider care plan.

Motivational interviewing

This approach is often used when working with people who have a substance misuse problem, however can be a useful framework when working with people to make any change to their behaviour. It is underpinned by Prochaska and DiClemente's (1986) transtheoretical model of change which focuses on the service user's motivation or readiness to change. They define four stages, however it is acknowledged that people will often move back and forth between stages:

1. Precontemplation – no recognition of the problem and therefore see no reason to change.
2. Contemplation – recognition and thinking of the problem leading to an openness to exploring the possibility of change.
3. Determination and action – preparing to make and making changes.
4. Maintenance – sustaining change and preventing relapse.

Motivational interviewing aims to enable the service user to identify the discrepancy between their current behaviour and any goals or hopes they have for their future. It recognises that people who abuse substances are often ambivalent or in two minds about their wish to engage in the behaviour and their commitment to restrain from the behaviour. Motivational interviewing techniques attempt to elicit and encourage the person's commitment to change by identifying factors which trigger the behaviour and exploring the consequences of engaging in the behaviour (Miller & Rollnick 1991).

Adopting this approach will require you to take a proactive and neutral position, often playing the role of the devil's advocate. Lecturing or attempting to advise the service user is thought to lead to further resistance to change and defensiveness. Therefore it is advisable to start with a behaviour that the person wants to change and emphasise their responsibility within the change process.

At each stage of the model, specific approaches or interventions may be relevant and Table 10.2 summarises these.

Table 10.2 Interventions to support change	
Precontemplation	Engagement and building of a therapeutic alliance which enables the service user to recognise the value of being involved with the service and establish their trust in the practitioner
	Gathering information on the person's readiness to change and the level of ambivalence they are expressing
Contemplation	Utilising the trusting relationship to explore the motivators for change
	Identifying the costs and benefits of change and costs and benefits of staying the same which are unique to that person
	Giving information on effects of their behaviour and reflect back aspects of their lifestyle which they appear to find problematic
	Negotiating short-term and realistic goals which are congruent with the person's readiness to change, e.g. reduction in the frequency or severity of the behaviour, avoidance of situations where behaviour is triggered, utilisation of an alternative behaviour which has a similar effect

Table 10.2 Interventions to support change—cont'd	
Action	Setting longer term goals which will enable sustainable behaviour change, e.g. making permanent changes to lifestyle which remove trigger factors, using prescribed medication to allow for reduction or removal of a substance by managing withdrawal effects, engaging with self-help groups for peer support and encouragement Adopting alternative coping skills which replace the behaviour or enable the service user to cope with short-term distress arising from the behaviour change Planning for achievement of positive goals for the future which are dependent on the successful behaviour change
Maintenance	Relapse prevention involving the identification of potential triggers which may lead to previous behaviours, coping skills, sources of support and contingency plans (see section in this chapter) Recognising achievements made and building on successes

Working with families

Involving families and informal carers in the care of service users has been highly advocated by research and policy (Department of Health (DH) 1999, Gamble & Brennan 2000, DH 2006, Mental Health Foundation 2010). The assessment of carers' needs is also a required element of the Care Programme Approach. This section aims to outline the skills and challenges of working with families.

This type of intervention should be distinguished from family therapy or family work. These are more specialist interventions which require specific qualifications and are often learnt and mastered under expert supervision.

Research suggests that the family can be highly facilitative in the recovery process due to the following reasons:
- They hold a deep knowledge of those they are in the relationship with, including their past history and developmental progress.
- They can help recognise early warning signs.
- They provide natural sources of emotional support.

However, families often report feeling that their personal needs are neglected by mental health services and their views and opinions are dismissed. The complex area of confidentiality is repeatedly recognised as a constraint to working with families. This is because the mental health practitioner has a duty to maintain the service user's confidentiality unless there are concerns regarding safety. Families can feel that confidentiality is used as an excuse to justify poor communication or reluctance to share information. It is important to explain the limitations of confidentiality to the family and to establish with the service user what information they are comfortable with being shared. This should be clearly documented to ensure that all members of the team respect the service user's wishes.

Despite this constraining factor, it is important to acknowledge the potential effects of learning that a loved one has a mental health problem and the consequent impact this will have on their future relationship. This might include the following feelings:
- Scared of the service user's behaviour and the implications of them receiving a psychiatric diagnosis.

- Sad or hopeless about how the mental health problems may impact on their life or influence their future.
- Guilty about the role they may have played in the development of the mental health problem.
- Angry with mental health services or in disagreement with their judgements.
- Bewildered, particularly if the person has no previous experience of mental health problems or services.
- Powerless to improve the situation.
- Isolated as a result of stigma experienced from communities, friends and other family members.
- Overprotective of the service user and highly focused on getting their needs met by services.

The consequence of this may be the development of their own mental health problems or a fractious beginning to relationships with mental health practitioners. These feelings will also potentially have an impact on the service user's relationship with the family member. The relationship is in danger of breaking down as the service user may feel blamed for the family's problems, a burden or a disappointment. Additionally, the service user may believe that they are held back by family members who doubt their potential in light of their mental health problems or who are reluctant to allow them to take risks. This type of reaction has been described as high expressed emotion and is characterised by critical comments and hostility towards service users or overinvolvement in their lives. Consider the following scenarios.

Overinvolvement

You are on placement with a nurse practitioner in a GP's surgery. You have been seeing Mary for a number of sessions due to her tearfulness and hopelessness. Her husband, Bob, insists on bringing her to the sessions and waits for her to finish, often coming in at the end of the session to ask if

she is getting better. At the last session Bob tells you he is seriously considering giving up work to look after his wife full time.

Critical comments and hostility

You are on placement at a residential rehabilitation unit. You answer the phone to Peter's sister who is complaining about her brother's personal hygiene. She is angry with staff for not assisting him to wash, dress and shave before his visit home. She tells you that she has sent him back to the unit and told him that he smells disgusting and is an embarrassment to the family.

Critical comments and hostility

You are on placement with a community mental health team. Your mentor is a community psychiatric nurse working with John, a 54-year-old man who lives at home with his elderly mother. When you visit his mother, she answers the door and immediately complains about her son.

'You just ask him what he's been up to this week.'

'I don't know how I can carry on putting up with him.'

'He's useless and does nothing to help.'

Activity

For the examples above, consider how you may respond:

1. Immediately.
2. In the longer term to improve the relationship.

The aim of working with families and informal carers is to address these types of reactions by supporting the family to express warmth towards the person who is experiencing mental health problems and develop positive coping strategies. This is known as low expressed emotion and is conducive to recovery.

> **Activity**
>
> 1. In your experience and observations of mental health practice, how have families or informal carers:
>   a. helped the person in their recovery?
>   b. hindered the person in their recovery?
> 2. For the examples you have identified, what evidence was there of high or low expressed emotion?
> 3. Discuss these examples with your mentor and identify how you might help to address the negative impact of high expressed emotion on the individual.

In order to help sustain relationships with families and carers, mental health practitioners can provide support and education. They may also open lines of communication between the service user and the family members to develop coping strategies, identify and solve problems. This is with the overall aim of maintaining or improving the relationships which the service user values. The structure and focus of the intervention will depend on the service user's and family's needs. An informal approach to giving support and information will be appropriate in many circumstances (Askey et al 2007). However, in situations where there is evidence of high expressed emotion or problems which are significantly affecting the service user's wellbeing, the following stages can provide the basis for facilitating this type of intervention. It is advisable that you work with your mentor to identify this need and discuss the contribution you can make to the intervention.

Stage 1: engaging families
- Consider with the service user who should be involved.
- Agree with the service user what information they are comfortable with being shared and discussed within interactions with family members.
- Offer positive, pleasant and consistent contact to family members.
- Show appropriate care and concern for the family situation.
- Speak to family members individually to gain their individual perspective on the situation and assess their level of understanding in relation to mental health problems.

Stage 2: setting the scene
- Find a convenient time and place to meet.
- Identify and agree upon the general purpose of the meetings. For example:
  - to share information and discuss the varied understanding of the mental health problems (this is sometimes described as psychoeducation)
  - to improve communication and understanding of each other's perspectives within the family
  - to solve problems which are impacting on the service user's wellbeing and recovery.
- Collaboratively set ground rules which will guide the group discussion. These might include the following.
  - each person will be given the opportunity to contribute to every discussion
  - we will agree to listen to and consider all views which are expressed
  - we will agree to address people directly and to not talk about someone while they are there
  - we will identify specific areas for change and commit to trying out possible solutions even if we are sceptical of the outcome.

Stage 3: identifying and addressing areas of concern (a problem-solving approach)
- Start by specifying in detail what the problem is.
- Identify everyone's view of the problem, particularly that of the service user.

- Enable people to state how the problem makes them feel.
- Elicit possible solutions from everyone.
- Look at the pros and cons of each possible solution.
- Compromise and agree on a desirable solution.
- Anticipate any obstacles.
- Identify clearly the action that needs to be taken, a timeline for when it should be achieved and the responsibilities of the people contributing in order for it to be achieved.
- Review progress and revise action at the next meeting.

Facilitating these types of interactions can be challenging for the mental health practitioner and it may be advisable to broach complex family situations in pairs to enable the effective management of potential dynamics or strong emotional reactions. It is important to focus upon the service user's voice within interaction in order to ensure that they are not used as a forum for further criticism or blame. This may require the mental health practitioner to take a more assertive approach at times depending on the personalities involved. The following are a number of hints and tips which can help when facilitating this type of discussion:

- Avoid jargon – this may exclude people from contributing to the discussion as they may not understand.
- Acknowledge expertise – recognise that the service user and family have understanding and information which is valuable to the process as a result of their lived experiences.
- Acknowledge loss – recognise how the person's experience of mental health problems has impacted on their lives and the adjustments which have had to be made as a result of this.
- Focus on strengths – identify positive elements of the relationship which are valued, recognise coping strategies which are already in place and goals for the future.

- Start with small problems which can be easily achieved to enable early success and establish a commitment to the process.
- Address critical comments directly and explore how they make the recipient feel.
- Attempt to identify what is underpinning the critical comment by considering the emotions which may be fuelling it, e.g. fear, guilt, frustration.
- Role model understanding and acceptance within the group.
- Be conscious of alliances you are making with individuals as this may influence your facilitation approach.

Relapse prevention

Relapse prevention refers to a set of interventions which aim to identify the early signs of relapse and act upon them to avoid the breakdown of mental health or minimise the negative impact of crisis on the individual's life (Birchwood et al 1989, van Meijel et al 2002a,b). It is a collaborative process where service users are viewed as the experts of their experience through the acknowledgment of personal strategies, skills and resources for self-management.

There are a number of relapse prevention tools, however they will commonly include the following:

1. Engagement and education –the Stress Vulnerability Model can be used to aid this process and the leaky bucket analogy described in Chapter 3 can be a helpful analogy.
2. Developing a relapse signature – identifying early warning signs of relapse.
3. Developing a relapse drill – agreeing and recording in advance the nature and timing of actions which should be followed if early warning signs are present.
4. Monitoring of the early warning signs and rehearsal of the relapse drill.

The Wellness Recovery Action Plan (WRAP) is a simple self-help system which facilitates the identification of personal resources and encourages people who experience mental distress to use these personal resources to stay well and help themselves during difficult periods. It is an example of a relapse prevention tool and was developed by Mary Ellen Copland who maintains that people with mental health issues can have hope, control over their lives, develop self-directed wellness plans and recover by working toward meeting their own life dreams and goals. These strategies and skills are being used worldwide both by individuals independently of support from mental health services and as part of approaches utilised within mental health services to promote recovery. You can hear Mary Ellen speak about the approach at http://www.mentalhealthrecovery.com and access the tools and supporting self-help resources that she has developed in collaboration with others who have experienced mental health problems.

The aim of WRAP is to give the person more control over their problems. The WRAP can become a practical support for recovery which can be referred to daily, as a reminder and guide, and also turned to at times of difficulty. It is designed as an aid for helping people to learn about themselves, what helps and what doesn't, and how to get progressively more in control of their life and experience of mental health issues. It also includes instructions on developing a crisis plan as a means of guiding others on how best to make decisions for the person during times when problems and symptoms have made it difficult for the person to do this for themselves.

A WRAP includes the following:

Developing a wellness toolbox: This involves the person asking themselves questions which help them to identify their personal resources, the values that underpin their beliefs and their hopes and goals for their future.

Evolving a daily maintenance plan: This will include a baseline description of how the person feels when they are well. This is important because this will differ for every individual. It is therefore essential not to judge a person's presentation on what you define as being well as the person may never have those feelings or describe themselves in that way. For example, some people may appear to be speaking quickly, finding it difficult to concentrate or sit still. This may be normal for them or part of their character and can be described as their premorbid personality. For some people, these ways of communicating are a sign that their mental health is deteriorating and are also known as early warning signs or prodromal symptoms.

Student reminders

It will be difficult for you to judge if a person's thoughts, feelings or behaviours are 'normal' for them when you first meet. Many students are surprised at how people can hold strange beliefs or behave in odd ways and still live very contented lives.

- Where a person has a WRAP or a relapse prevention plan, it can be helpful to read this before you meet the person as this will allow you to gain some awareness of how they describe themselves when they are feeling well.
- If this is not available, you may wish to ask your mentor for this information.
- Following your contact with the person, talk with your mentor about your observations of the person's thoughts, feelings and behaviour and how this compares with your preconceptions of what it means to be mentally well.

The daily maintenance plan will also include the things that the person does every day to help maintain and sustain their wellbeing and the things which they may have to do that they might find difficult.

An example could be opening post or making a phone call. Additionally the tool encourages people to think about the things that help them but that they are less likely to do when they are finding their mental health is negatively affecting them. For example, some people find contact with others helpful, however tend to withdraw or isolate themselves when feeling unwell. This can give you an insight into how you can encourage the person to do the things that help during difficult periods or provide support to enable them to maintain contact with others, even when this feels overwhelming.

Understanding triggers and what can be done about them

This section of the WRAP is about identifying the events or circumstances that are likely to trigger unhelpful or distressing thoughts or behaviours. The person identifies how they can avoid the trigger or looks at how they will cope with it if it does arise. It often helps to look back at previous periods of crisis and to think about what precipitated the difficulties and what the person or others did which was helpful or unhelpful during that time.

Identifying early warning signs (relapse drill)

Early warning signs are the subtle changes in thoughts, feelings and behaviours which can indicate to the person or others that action needs to be taken to prevent the difficulties getting worse. For example, some people might have increasing feelings of low motivation and appear more reluctant to care for themselves. Others may start to spend lots of money and not worry about the consequences in a way which is out of character. In some cases, people can become easily agitated or fearful for their safety which may result in unusual behaviour.

It is important that the person and those around them are able to recognise these changes and identify what action can be taken to help. This may include increased support from family, friends or mental health services, reducing unnecessary stress, engaging in activities which help to relieve stress and reviewing medication.

You can facilitate the identification of early warning signs in the following ways:

1. Time line – this is a detailed account of the person's account of the events and experiences leading up to previous relapses. It enables the identification of factors that had an impact on the onset of relapse in the past.
2. Card sort exercise – the service user identifies early warning signs using cards which state common signs of relapse. They then arrange them into early, middle and late signs of relapse or signs which are constant during periods of stress.
3. Review information from both exercises with close family/friends to identify gaps that the service user finds difficult to remember.

These signs can be monitored both directly and indirectly. To directly monitor the signs, the person may score the degree to which they are experiencing the sign on a scale of 1 to 10. To indirectly monitor the signs, the service user, family and mental health practitioner can be aware if circumstances or life changes which have led to relapse in the past reoccur, in order to closely monitor their impact.

Signs that things are breaking down

This section asks the person to identify how they think, feel and behave when the situation has become very distressing, difficult to manage or dangerous. Often this is an extremely unpleasant experience for the person and they may need others to enable them to stop things getting worse, particularly if the person feels unable to identify or articulate their own needs at this time. It is therefore essential to agree in advance how the person would like to be supported during these times and the things that help reduce their distress. For example, some people find that particular environments are comforting and provide a level of security while others find similar environments frightening and stressful. There are certain medications which people may have found helpful in the past during periods of distress and others that they have found ineffective or that have negative side effects.

Crisis planning (relapse drill)
The crisis plan draws together all of this information to enable the person to communicate their views, wants and needs during periods of crisis. It should include the names and contacts of people who they would like to support their care during periods of crisis and those who they would not like involved. It should detail the interventions, treatments and care setting you find helpful, those which should be avoided and their reasons for this. Finally the crisis plan should identify when it should be deactivated and the person is able to take back personal control of their care by being included in decisions.

Postcrisis planning
The postcrisis plan emphasises that crisis is not a failure and does not mean that recovery is not possible for the person. It prompts the person to reflect on the experience and learn more about themselves in order to review the WRAP and identify what worked and what didn't.

It may be helpful to summarise this information for the service user, family and people involved in their care to access quickly. An example is given in Table 10.3.

Table 10.3 Example of summarised relapse prevention plan

Relapse signature	Relapse drill
1. Feel worried about what Cathy next door thinks of me	1. Talk to husband John and CPN Gemma about how I am feeling
2. Can't get to sleep at night	2. Challenge my thoughts about Cathy
3. Lose my temper with John	3. Watch TV to take my mind off my worries
4. Stay inside and don't see Cathy	4. Have a bath and listen to music
5. Hear my mum's voice talking about how nobody likes me	5. Talk to Gemma about visiting more often and medication options
6. Cut my arms to punish myself for being a horrid person	6. Contact crisis team for additional support when Gemma is not available

Emergency contact details

John Mobile – 07xxxxxxx
Gemma mobile – 07xxxxxxxx
Community Mental Health Team – 0155xxxxxx
Crisis and Home Treatment Team – 0155xxxxxxx

While there is evidence to support the value of relapse prevention, it can be challenging in some circumstances. For example, when identifying early warning signs, the service user may not agree with the perceptions of family members or mental health practitioners. This is because many people experience difficulty with structuring their own reality leading up to relapse. This is sometimes referred to as lack of insight and has the potential to cause friction if the memory of past relapse remains distressing for those involved. Taking a collaborative approach to relapse prevention can alleviate these issues. This may involve agreeing to disagree on some areas in order to ensure that each person's perspective has been considered.

Also some people cope with their mental health problem by 'sealing over'. This means they wish to forget previous crisis periods and are therefore unlikely to want to consider past experiences and the possibility of future relapse. It will be important in these circumstances to work at a pace that they are comfortable with. This might involve using approaches such as the card sort exercise which depersonalises the experience initially.

Finally the service user may experience feelings of guilt or hopelessness if they are proactive and engaged in relapse prevention strategies but relapse still occurs. In order to alleviate this issue, the mental health practitioner should emphasise that, while the person has control over their mental health and future relapse, it should not be considered as a failure and there is still value in limiting the negative impact that relapse has on a person's life.

References

Askey, R., Gamble, C., Gray, R., 2007. Family work in first-onset psychosis: a literature review. Journal of Psychiatric and Mental Health Nursing 14, 356–365.

Birchwood, M., Smith, J., MacMillan, F., et al., 1989. Predicting relapse in schizophrenia: the development of an early warning signs monitoring system using patients and families as observers. A preliminary investigation. Psychol. Med. 19, 649–656.

Department of Health, 1999. National service framework for mental health. HMSO, London.

Department of Health, 2006. From values to action: Chief Nursing Officer's review of mental health nurse education. HMSO, London.

Gamble, C., Brennan, G., 2000. Working with families and informal carers. In: Gamble, C., Brennan, G. (Eds.), Working with serious mental illness: a manual for clinical practice. Baillière Tindall, London.

Miller, W.R., Rollnick, S., 1991. Motivational interviewing: preparing people to change addictive behaviours. Guilford Press, New York.

Mills, J., 2006. Dealing with voices and strange thoughts. In: Gamble, C., Brennan, G. (Eds.), Working with serious mental illness: a manual for clinical practice. Baillière Tindall, London.

Prochaska, J.O., DiClemente, C.C., 1986. Transtheoretical therapy: towards a comprehensive model of change. In: Miller, W., Heather, N. (Eds.), Treating addictive behaviours: process of change. Plenum Press, New York.

Mental Health Foundation, 2010. The lonely society. MHF, London.

van Meijel, B., van der Gaag, M., Khan, R.S., Grypdonck, M., 2002a. The practice of early recognition and early intervention to prevent psychotic relapse in patients with schizophrenia: an exploratory study. Part 1. Journal of Psychiatric and Mental Health Nursing 9, 347–355.

van Meijel, B., van der Gaag, M., Khan, R.S., Grypdonck, M., 2002b. The practice of early recognition and early intervention to prevent psychotic relapse in patients with schizophrenia: an exploratory study. Part 2. Journal of Psychiatric and Mental Health Nursing 9, 357–363.

Zubin, J., Spring, B., 1977. Vulnerability: a new view on schizophrenia. Journal of Abnormal Psychology 86, 103–126.

Further reading

Phillips, P., Callaghan, P., 2009. Working with people with substance misuse problems. In: Callaghan, P., Playle, J., Cooper, L. (Eds.), Mental health nursing skills. Oxford University Press, New York.

Treasure, J., 2004. Motivational interviewing. Advances in Psychiatric Treatment 10, 331–337.

11

Working with people who are anxious or low in mood

CHAPTER AIMS

- To describe the Five Areas model of assessment and formulation
- To describe a series of psychological interventions, underpinned by a cognitive behavioural therapy approach, which aim to:
  - challenge unhelpful thinking styles
  - overcome reduced activity
  - overcome increased anxiety
- To identify how these interventions might be applied to your mental health nursing practice

Introduction

The interventions and clinical skills described in this chapter are informed by a cognitive behavioural therapy (CBT) approach (see Ch. 3). There is a growing evidence base for the effectiveness of these interventions when working with people who are anxious or low in mood. Additionally there has been strong political support to increase access to psychological interventions in the UK which has led to investment in specific training and service

programmes (Department of Health 2008). Efforts have been made to identify the positive elements of a CBT approach and adapt them so that a greater number of practitioners can feel confident using them in mainstream mental health practice. The interventions described here utilise these adaptations and are reflective of the contemporary ways in which CBT is delivered in mainstream services. More information and resources on this approach can be found at http://www.fiveareas.com/resourcearea/ (accessed June 2011). Specialist services do still exist where experienced CBT therapists adopt more traditional approaches and work with people with complex problems.

The interventions described here attempt to improve anxiety and low mood by influencing the way a person perceives and responds to specific situations. This involves conducting a thorough assessment which identifies how a recent life situation alters thinking, behaviour, emotional and physical feelings and how these areas impact on each other to lead to a problematic response. Interventions will commonly focus on changing one of these areas as a way of breaking unhelpful cycles of thoughts, feelings and behaviours. This is based on the fundamental principle of CBT which maintains that what people think affects how they feel emotionally and physically and consequently what they do. Interventions are often short term and tend to focus on a specific problem in the here and now as opposed to past life events which have contributed to the person's current issues. As a student on a mental health placement, you could be involved in delivering an intervention underpinned by this approach.

The Five Areas assessment model

The Five Areas assessment model recognises that when people are feeling anxious or low in mood their thinking can become extreme and unhelpful. For example, people may see themselves as worthless or incompetent which then leads to reduced or avoidant behaviours. The model identifies five domains within which a person's problematic thinking and behaviour can be examined, and the links between each area can be established (Williams & Garland 2002a):

1. Life situation, relationships and practical problems.
2. Altered thinking.
3. Altered emotions (mood or feelings).
4. Altered physical feelings.
5. Altered behaviour or activity levels.

Focused and specific questions are asked to explore the problematic life situation and ascertain how it is impacting on or being maintained by the remaining four areas. For example:

Area 2: altered thinking
- How do you see yourself?
- How do others see you?

Area 3: altered emotions
- How would you describe your mood?
- How has this changed?
- How would you feel about ...? (Describe specific scenarios to ascertain the emotional response, e.g. fearful, angry, guilty or embarrassed.)

Area 4: altered physical symptoms
- How would you describe your sleep, appetite, concentration, energy levels, etc.?
- How easy do you find it to relax?
- How would you describe the feelings in your muscles?

Area 5: altered behaviour
- What things have you stopped doing since you have been feeling this way?
- What things have you started doing to help you cope with the way you have been feeling?

(For a more extensive list of example questions, see Williams & Garland 2002a.)

This approach to assessment aims to inform interventions by identifying clear target areas for change, as making alterations in any one of the domains of the Five Areas model is assumed to lead to improvements in other areas. The model can easily be understood by service users and enables them to recognise their own patterns of thoughts and behaviours from a more objective position. Together the mental health practitioner and the service user can identify how the problem is maintained by specific thoughts, feelings and behaviours which allows them to see the potential for improvement.

The information gathered from the assessment process is summarised under the five domains in a diagram which identifies the relationship between the areas. This can be used to feed back to the multidisciplinary team so that the whole team can gain an understanding of the person's problems and adopt a consistent approach to interventions. An example of when this could be particularly helpful would be if a service user is coping with anxiety through seeking constant reassurance. You may be working with them to change this behaviour and will require other members of the team to support this intervention by not giving reassurance when the service user requests it.

Once the assessment is complete, a plan for intervention is agreed by identifying the area which is likely to have the most significant impact on the defined problem. The following interventions are examples of approaches which are commonly adopted in mental health practice.

Challenging unhelpful thinking styles

The thinking style associated with a problem or behaviour will often become extreme or unhelpful if a person is experiencing anxiety or low mood. You may hear this referred to as negative automatic thoughts, thinking errors or cognitive distortions. They tend to be consistent and lead to misinterpretation of everyday situations. There are common unhelpful thinking styles which lead people to blow issues out of proportion or downplay their ability to cope with a problem. These could include the following:

- A high level of self-criticism.
- A negative attitude towards past and current events.
- Negative predictions about the future.
- Presuming others think badly of them without evidence to suggest that this is the case.
- Feeling responsible for poor outcomes.
- Taking feedback as criticism and personalising criticism which is not directly related to them.
- Holding high standards for self which are likely to be impossible to meet.

It is important to recognise that we all hold some unhelpful thinking styles and you may be able to apply some of the examples given above to yourself at times. These tend to become problematic when these thoughts become frequent and hard to dismiss which then leads to significant levels of distress.

In the following scenario, try to identify the unhelpful thinking styles which are present.

Case history

Jane is a 38-year-old single woman who lives alone in a small flat and works as a legal secretary. She has been seeing her doctor for several months complaining of lack of appetite, feeling listless and no longer enjoying her work. After extensive tests revealed no physical health problems, her GP referred her to a psychiatrist for assessment. Although initially reluctant, Jane eventually agreed. The psychiatrist diagnosed Jane with mild depression and prescribed a course of antidepressant medication. Jane was reluctant to take the tablets and enquired whether there was any alternative. She was told about cognitive behavioural therapy which she chose to take up.

During the first meetings, Jane spoke about always feeling different and isolated from other people but things had become worse over the past few months following a date with a work colleague. Jane had never got on well with men and could see nothing in herself that men would find attractive. She had therefore resigned herself to remaining single and had arranged her life accordingly. When a colleague asked her out for a meal, she was flattered and immediately agreed. However, on reflection, she felt her decision had been hasty and was convinced he had only asked her out of pity. Her doubts were confirmed on the date when she acted clumsily and could think of nothing interesting to say. The next day at work her colleague made no attempt to ask her out again. Since that time Jane had found it difficult to talk to men and women. She felt her work colleagues were talking about her behind her back and that she was completely unlikable. She had also lost her desire to play her piano in the local church which was her main hobby.

Activity

While on placement you should try to identify these thinking styles among the service users you are working with. You may also be able to recognise them within yourself and friends and family.

Stage 1: recognising unhelpful thinking styles

Interventions which aim to challenge unhelpful thinking styles start with helping the service user to recognise them, identify the impact they have on how they feel and what they do as a response. The follow steps will guide you through this process:

1. Use the list above (p. 165) to talk about if and when the service user has noticed adopting any of these thinking styles.
2. Ask the person to describe the general situations or events when they noticed the thinking style was present. Examples might include:
   a. a job interview
   b. a friend not phoning back when they have left a message
   c. a high level of disappointment with feedback from colleagues despite it being predominantly positive.
3. Observe how the person's mood changes while describing the situation and ask them to discuss their current thoughts in relation to the event and how it is making them feel to talk about it.

Stage 2: investigating the thinking style

4. Ask the service user to identify a recent situation where they have felt highly distressed and explore this in depth by considering:
   a. the time, place, people present, content and context of the event
   b. the emotional and physical feelings which were present
   c. the severity of these feelings. They may find it helpful to rate these on a scale of 1 to 10

d. the thinking styles which were present when emotion levels were at their highest
e. how the thought was experienced, e.g. as a statement in their head, a colour, an image from their perspective or from another person's perspective
f. their conviction in the thought. They may also find it helpful to rate this on a scale of 1 to 10.

5. Identify together the link between the emotional and physical feelings and the thinking style.
6. Discuss what the service user did to relieve their distress and consider if this involved further unhelpful thinking styles.

(Adapted from Williams & Garland 2002b.)

 Activity

Before you initiate exploring unhelpful thinking styles with a service user, it is beneficial to consider how you might respond to the questions above based on an event when you have noticed your mood altering. Once you have completed this exercise, consider the following:

1. What did you find challenging about this exercise?
2. How did you find remembering the details of the event or situation?
3. How did you find describing the distressing experience?
4. How did you find distinguishing your thoughts from your feelings?

Discuss with your mentor what you have learnt from completing the task yourself and how this might impact on the way you would broach this with a service user?

Stage 3: challenging unhelpful thinking styles

Once the service user is well practised at identifying their unhelpful thinking styles and is aware of them in day-to-day situations, you can then move onto approaches which challenge them. This is with the view to altering the way a person perceives a situation which will impact on their emotional and behavioural response. This approach is similar to that described in Chapter 13 for testing unusual beliefs and involves encouraging the person to focus on the most emotion-inducing thought (sometimes referred to as the 'hot thought') and considering the evidence which supports and challenges their conviction in it.

Williams and Garland (2002b) suggest the following questions can be helpful prompts for facilitating this process:

Reasons supporting the immediate thought

- List all the reasons why I believed the immediate thought at the time.

Evidence against the immediate thought

- Is there anything to make me think the thought is incorrect?
- Are there any other ways of explaining the situation that are more accurate?
- If I wasn't feeling like this, what would I say?
- Would I tell a friend who believed the same thought that they were wrong?
- What would other people say?
- Have others given me different opinions about the thought?

Based on the service user's response to these questions, you can then work together to identify a more balanced conclusion to the thought and consider what can be changed to reinforce the balanced perspective and undermine the unhelpful or extreme immediate response. This change should allow the person to test out the balanced conclusion in everyday life in order to increase their evidence against the immediate thought. It will also move the intervention to a practical task which the person is able to complete outside of the session. Evidence suggests that this is an important aspect of embedding change into day-to-day life.

If we consider the case study above describing Jane's unhelpful thinking styles, the types of changes she might consider would be based upon challenging her thoughts around how others perceive her. Therefore she would need to start by identifying the evidence for and against the thought in order to come to a more balanced conclusion. For example, Jane may conclude that her perceptions of her work colleagues are unfounded because she noticed them respond differently to her immediately and therefore they could not have known how the meal had gone. In order to test this conclusion, she may consider:

- Initiating a conversation with a work colleague to see how they respond to her.
- Confiding in a friend or colleague about her perception of the meal and asking how they might have perceived the gentleman's response the next day.
- Requesting feedback from friends or colleagues on what they value about her during informal conversation.

The outcome of the change should be discussed in depth and may involve further identification and challenge of unhelpful thoughts. The testing of unhelpful thoughts will inevitably be a difficult prospect particularly if the person is more inclined to avoid confronting the situation. It is important to recognise that change is hard and is likely to involve some discomfort. However, the therapeutic relationship can provide the safe environment for a person to take these steps provided that they are clear about the rationale and in agreement with aims of the intervention.

Overcoming reduced activity

The impact of low mood on thoughts and feelings is often a decrease in activity. This is due to a combination of unhelpful thought patterns, low energy levels and a lack in feelings of pleasure, achievement or enjoyment. This can impact on the person's day-to-day functioning as initially pleasurable activities become less of a priority and eventually essential tasks become overwhelming. The social isolation which can result from this leads to a loss of support or limits access to help from friends, family or healthcare professionals.

Interventions which aim to address decreased activity involve developing a step-by-step plan of reintroducing aspects of a person's life that they previously enjoyed or are necessary for day-to-day functioning (Martell et al 2001, Hopko et al 2003). This type of intervention is commonly known as behavioural activation. The steps outlined below are a brief introduction to behavioural activation and can inform your approach to working with service users who have decreased activity levels.

Step 1

Discuss the rationale for the intervention and ensure the service user has a clear understanding of the theory which underpins it. It may be helpful to use the Five Areas model to aid this process.

Step 2

Identify how the person is currently coping with their low mood or anxiety. For example, are they:
- decreasing their activity
- avoiding situations
- adopting unhelpful safety behaviours which provide distraction, reassurance, artificially blocking of emotion or a release of emotions.

It is likely that this behaviour is acting to reinforce or maintain the problem and therefore can become the target for intervention. This information can be gathered by general conversation or by asking the person to keep an activity diary recording what they did, where the activity took place, when they did it and who they did it with, over a 1-week period. This can be a challenging task for people who are experiencing low motivation and may reinforce the perception that they are achieving very little or engaging in limited activities that they enjoy. A person's response to completing the diary will provide valuable information and will often require a level of encouragement and reassurance.

Step 3

Identify activities that the service user would like to do. These may be activities that they have reduced or given up since they have experienced a change in mood. Once these activities have been listed, they should be categorised into routine, pleasurable and necessary.

Step 4

Organise the list into order of difficulty under the headings most difficult, medium difficulty and easiest. Items from each of the categories above should be included under each of the headings to ensure that activities that are necessary but most difficult are addressed. An example of how this might look is given in Table 11.1.

Step 5

Plan to implement some of the activities identified from each of the categories. Start with the easiest, small and regular activities which can provide quick success and increased motivation to tackle the more challenging activities. A specific plan should be devised to ensure that the service user is clear about what activity is scheduled, when, where and who with. The person's activity should then be recorded in a dairy to enable

Table 11.1 Example of behavioural activation chart

	Routine	Pleasurable	Necessary
Most difficult	Answering the phone	Going to the gym	Looking for a new job Shopping for food
Medium difficulty	Cooking the kids a dinner with fresh ingredients Cleaning the house	Watching a film Concentrating on what my kids are telling me about their day	Paying the bills on time Picking the kids up from school
Easiest	Making the bed Loading the dishwasher	Reading a magazine	Getting up in the morning

you both to assess the success of the plan and review it in order to set new goals.

Step 6
Jointly review the achievements in relation to the planned activity under each of the categories. Within the review, you should identify successes, problem solve any barriers to putting plans into action and discuss avoidant behaviours when plans have not been followed through.

Step 7
A return to decreased activity can occur if the person's mood drops further or they do not feel the longer term benefits of their increased activity. Supporting the person to identify early warning signs of decreased activity can help with preventing relapse. It is also essential to discuss the person's expectation of the impact of the intervention. This will involve normalising their responses and reinforcing the service user's achievements. It is unrealistic to assume that they will always feel motivated to complete necessary tasks or that pleasurable activities will always meet their expectations. Therefore it may be helpful to discuss how their reaction is similar to other people who are not experiencing a mental health problem.

A problem-solving approach has also been advocated as a way of addressing decreased activity levels (Garland et al 2002). In the case study above describing Jane, this will involve considering the stages in Table 11.2.

The example given in the table represents a positive outcome arising from a collaborative and well-planned approach. However, if the outcome had been less successful, it could still provide valuable learning and should not be viewed as a failure. The reasons why the plan did not go well can be discussed and a revised plan can be devised which takes into account unforeseen challenges or barriers.

The success arising from this behaviour change is likely to give Jane increased motivation to address other areas of decreased activity and continue to work towards her longer term goals. Applying the same principles will enable her to become practised at approaching problems in this way. In a problem-solving approach it is important to move at a pace that the service user is comfortable with while encouraging them to continually build upon achievements and move forward. This may involve rating the specific problems and broaching the ones which initially feel least challenging and setting time scales for when to address each area.

Table 11.2 Example of a problem-solving approach to addressing reduced activity levels

Problem-solving approach	Example		Note
1. Identify one behaviour to change	Start playing the piano again at church for the Sunday service		This represents an activity which previously gave Jane pleasure but that has become low priority as a result of her mood
2. Brainstorm possible solutions	1. Play for a short period of time on my own 2. Play one piece at church which I know well and comes easily to me 3. Play in the Sunday service where there are lots of people		This may be challenging for Jane as a result of her mental health difficulties. You should reinforce that all suggestions are valid and offer potential suggestions if she is struggling
3. Look for the advantages and disadvantages of each option	Advantages 1. This would get me started and remind me what I am missing 2. This would be quite easy as I wouldn't need to concentrate too much 3. This would throw me in at the deep end – sink or swim I suppose	Disadvantages 1. I don't get as much pleasure from playing alone and would still miss seeing people at church 2. It is a little bit scary as I might make a mistake 3. I would feel really worried about this as I am out of practice and I'm sure people would think I am rubbish	Option 1 represents the continued avoidance of the activity and, while it could be a good start, it is unlikely to have the outcome that Jane is looking for Option 3 may lead to a negative outcome as it could be overwhelming for Jane and could reinforce Jane's unhelpful thoughts Option 2 is realistic and is most likely to succeed. It can also be implemented in the short term and is therefore practical

Table 11.2 Example of a problem-solving approach to addressing reduced activity levels—cont'd

Problem-solving approach	Example	Note
4. Choose a solution	Play a piece at church which I know well and comes easily to me	You should work with Jane to identify which option is the most desirable and likely to work towards the target change that you are both aiming for
5. Plan the steps to implement the solution	1. Select a piece of music that I feel comfortable with playing 2. Practice playing the piece in my own home 3. Persevere if I do not master the piece straight away 4. Contact the vicar and offer to play at next Thursday's service 5. Arrive early to get myself settled and clarify when I will be playing during the service 6. Think about my thoughts and feelings during the process and attempt to dismiss my unhelpful thoughts	Support Jane to identify what she is going to do and when she is going to do it. It may be helpful to write this down as memory can be effected by mental health problems
6. Carry out the change	When practising the piece, Jane becomes nervous about playing in public and makes mistakes. She thinks that she is hopeless and seriously considers not contacting the vicar to volunteer to play. However, she returns to her plan and reminds herself to persevere. She eventually plays it through without making any mistakes which undermines her unhelpful thought and gives her confidence to contact the vicar	Identify the positive elements and acknowledge the achievement she has made
7. Review the outcome of the change	Jane feels that the change went well. Although she did find the performance challenging, the vicar and members of the congregation told her they had missed her playing and have enjoyed having her back	Discuss with Jane what she has learnt from making the change and how she feels it went. This success provides the opportunity to consider how it will contribute to the achievement of Jane's original long-term target change

Overcoming increased anxiety

If a situation is feared, the body will increase levels of adrenaline to help us be alert and responsive to a potential threat. This leads to physical symptoms such as increased heart rate and hyperventilation. This response is commonly known as flight, fight or freeze. Once we feel safe again, the body calms our reactions down and helps us to return to a balanced state.

The most common approach used for helping people to overcome increased anxiety is known as exposure. This is based on the assumption that the more we expose ourselves to anxiety-provoking situations, the more able we are to cope with them. People with increased levels of anxiety will often fear everyday situations such as going to the supermarket or getting on the bus. This may be due to an unhelpful thinking pattern which is underpinning this fear or a misinterpretation of the physical symptoms of anxiety as potentially life threatening. When faced with a feared situation, the person is likely to experience anxiety almost immediately. The body experiences unpleasant physical sensations such as nausea or excess sweating that make the person feel weak. In response to these sensations the person will often attempt to leave (flight) to relieve the anxiety and physical sensations.

Alternatively, when a person is anxious they tend to avoid situations which they perceive as potentially anxiety provoking. Avoidance can be effective in the short term, however in the long term it can lead to an increased and more generalised anxiety as the person's confidence is undermined and their level of activity becomes more and more restricted. This is supported by behavioural theory described in Chapter 3. It can also maintain unhelpful thoughts as the person is not placing themselves in situations where their thoughts can be challenged.

According to conditional learning theory (described in Ch. 3), the best way to respond to these sensations is to stay in the situation long enough for the body to get used to it and to feel safe enough to let the anxiety levels drop. This will teach the body that the situation does not need to be feared and undermine the unhelpful thinking patterns which are contributing to maintaining the problematic response.

The prospect of staying in the situation may feel too challenging for some people and therefore a step-by-step approach may be helpful. This is often known as graded exposure. This requires the service user to define their overall target goal and then to identify related tasks which they can complete which will enable them to gradually develop their resilience to the feared situation. This should start with the least feared option and build up to the most feared. Some people find it helpful to rate these on a scale of 1 to 10. For example:

Most feared:
- Getting on the bus during busy periods (10/10).
- Getting on the bus during quieter periods (8/10).
- Standing at the bus stop (5/10).
- Walking to the bus stop (4/10).

Least feared:
- Leaving the house and walking to the end of the road (3/10).

An alternative approach is known as habituation and involves staying in the anxiety-provoking situation for gradually increasing periods of time. This is particularly helpful if the person believes that their physical symptoms will continue to get worse and may lead to highly distressing outcomes such as fainting, wetting themselves or having a heart attack. The person should be encouraged to rate their anxiety levels during the period of time spent in the situation in order to map the peaks and recognise their increased resilience over time.

The problem-solving approach advocated by Garland et al (2002) can also be adopted for addressing avoidance or unhelpful safety behaviours arising from feelings of anxiety. Table 11.3 considers Selena's problem with drinking alcohol arising from her attempts to cope with the anxiety she experiences when in the supermarket.

Table 11.3 Example of problem-solving approach to addressing increased anxiety

Problem-solving approach	Example		Note
Identify one behaviour to change	Drinking a bottle of wine before going to the shops to chill me out and block out my thoughts		This represents an unhelpful safety behaviour as it artificially blocks the emotional and physical response and can lead to alcohol dependency as a coping strategy
Brainstorm possible solutions	1. Don't have a drink and see what happens 2. Drink a glass of wine instead of a bottle 3. Travel to the shop with a friend and ask her to wait outside 4. Order shopping over the Internet 5. Talk to myself in my head to calm me down		This may be challenging for Selena as a result of her mental health difficulties. You should reinforce that all suggestions are valid and offer potential suggestions if she is struggling
Look for the advantages and disadvantages of each option	Advantages 1. Test out if what I think will happen will actually happen 2. I will still be aware of my thoughts and feelings 3. I will feel reassured by my friend being outside	Disadvantages 1. I feel worried and scared about giving it a go 2. I am still using something to block out my thoughts and feelings 3. If my friend can't make it I will feel more anxious in the long term	Options 2, 3, and 4 represent alternative safety behaviours and are unlikely to address the unhelpful thoughts and feelings in the longer term While option 1 represents the most challenging option, it is likely to impact most on Selena's overall target for change. She will be testing out her fears and allowing herself to discover that they are unhelpful and untrue

Continued

Table 11.3 Example of problem-solving approach to addressing increased anxiety—cont'd

Problem-solving approach	Example		Note
	4. I get my shopping and don't need a drink	4. I am avoiding the problem and won't ever be able to go to the shops	
Choose a solution	Don't have a drink and see what happens		You should work with Selena to identify which option is the most desirable and likely to work towards the target change that you are both aiming for
Plan the steps to implement the solution	1. Write a shopping list so I am prepared when I walk into the shop 2. Go shopping on Tuesday evening when it is moderately busy 3. Focus on the task and not on other people around me 4. If I start to feel anxious, stay in the shop and walk around slowly for 10 minutes 5. Take note of how I am feeling, what I am thinking and my level of anxiety		Support Selena to identify what she is going to do and when she is going to do it. It may be helpful to write this down as memory can be effected by mental health problems
Carry out the change	Selena goes to the shop prepared with her shopping list and at the time in her plan. However, as she is walking around the shop she finds herself walking quicker to get it done as soon as possible. Her eyesight becomes blurred and she is unable to see her shopping list. She leaves the shop within 7 minutes and without everything on her list.		Identify the positive elements and acknowledge the achievement she has made

Table 11.3 Example of problem-solving approach to addressing increased anxiety—cont'd

Problem-solving approach	Example	Note
Review the outcome of the change	Selena felt that the change went better than she expected as she was able to enter the supermarket without having had a drink beforehand. She identified that her anxiety levels went up when she began to walk faster and intends to try this again making a conscious effort to walk at a slower pace	In this case, elements of the plan were successful and it is important to acknowledge this. It can also provide a good opportunity to identify the thoughts and feeling which led to the increased anxiety and review the plan in accordance with this

It is important to identify if the person is adopting any safety behaviours to allow them to complete the task or stay in the situation without experiencing anxiety, as this will limit their exposure and prevent them from adapting to the response. For example, they might meet a friend to support them to walk to the bus stop or listen to music to distract themselves from the thoughts and physical sensations. While these may provide short-term relief, they will not address the target goal.

Each of these approaches are examples of behavioural experiments which can be carried out by the service user in between sessions. The outcome should be discussed in depth in order to review challenges, progress and continually move forward. It is also essential to identify how the evidence gained from the experiment is contributing to the evidence for and against the unhelpful thinking pattern and revisit the Five Areas assessment to consider how the associations between each area are influencing the person's progress.

References

Department of Health, 2008. Improving access to psychological therapies implementation plan: national guidelines for regional delivery. DH, London.

Garland, A., Fox, R., Williams, C., 2002. Overcoming reduced activity and avoidance: a Five Areas approach. Advances in Psychiatric Treatment 8, 453–462.

Hopko, D.R., Lejuez, C.W., Ruggiero, K.J., Eifert, G.H., 2003. Contemporary behavioural activation treatments for depression: procedures, principles and progress. Clinical Psychology Review 23, 699–717.

Martell, C., Addis, M., Jacobson, N., 2001. Depression in context. Strategies for guided action. Norton, New York.

Williams, C., Garland, A., 2002a. A cognitive-behavioural therapy assessment model for use in everyday clinical practice. Advances in Psychiatric Treatment 8, 172–179.

Williams, C., Garland, A., 2002b. Identifying and challenging unhelpful thinking. Advances in Psychiatric Treatment 8, 377–386.

Further reading

Richards, D., 2009. Behavioural activation. In: Callaghan, P., Playle, J., Cooper, L. (Eds.), Mental health nursing skills. Oxford University Press, New York.

Williams, C., 2001. Overcoming depression. Arnold, London.
Williams, C., Richards, P., Whitton, I., 2002. I'm not supposed to feel like this. Hodder and Stoughton, London.

Websites

Five Areas assessment information, http://www.fiveareas.com/resourcearea/index.php (accessed June 2011).

12   Assessing and managing risk

CHAPTER AIMS

- To develop understanding of risk assessment
- To identify skills and approaches to support effective risk assessment and management
- To develop understanding of positive risk taking
- To critically analyse risk in mental health practice
- To identify opportunities to and participate in risk assessment in mental health practice

Introduction

This chapter examines approaches that underpin risk assessment in contemporary mental health settings. It considers the skills that support good practice in risk assessment and management for mental health nurses and supports you to identify how you may learn about risk and contribute to risk assessment and management.

Risk assessment and management

Assessing and managing risk is an important skill within contemporary mental health nursing practice. Working with risk is a key feature of mental health policy (Department of Health (DH) 1999, DH 2006). It involves recognising, responding to and working with individuals to manage their own level of risk (DH 2004). It can also involve enabling people to take risks to work towards their recovery. This chapter examines risk in the context of mental health nursing practice and uses a scenario to help you explore this critically.

Risks in relation to mental health

Risk is most commonly understood in relation to the risks posed by people with mental health problems, either to themselves through self-harm, neglect or suicide or to others through violence. Identifying and assessing such risk is supported by a variety of risk assessment tools (examined briefly under the actuarial

---

◑ Reflection point

Think about the journey that you took to get to placement. Make a list of the risks that were present on that journey. It may help you to identify the following:

1. What were the potential threats or dangers?
2. How were these avoided?

While making this list, also have a think about any risks you took. It may help you to identify:

1. Were there any hazards that you overcame with a beneficial outcome?

After you have made a list, try and identify what skills you used to assess what risks you identified. Were some of the risks bigger or seen as more dangerous?

This exercise helps to identify that risk is part of everyday life for everyone (an issue that can be lost in the focus on risk in mental health practice). It also identifies and uses some skills which may inform your approach to risk assessment in mental health practice. This will be revisited in activities later in the chapter.

approach below). Within modern mental health services, professionals can often feel that their clinical abilities are judged by their ability to control and manage risk (Repper & Perkins 2003). This reflects the significant role risk has come to occupy within services. In order to understand this fully, it is important to consider the social and historical position of the concept of risk.

Following the advent of community care, people with mental health problems were more present within the community. Chapter 2 recognised that public perception of people with mental

health problems is often lacking in understanding. Community care further highlighted this perception towards mental illness. This was exacerbated by a number of high-profile incidents of violence perpetrated by people with mental health problems. The manner in which the media reported such incidents has been identified as perpetuating a link between violence and mental illness (Paterson & Stark 2001). This culminated in a situation where the government, media and sections of the public perceived care in the community had failed.

Following these incidents the government introduced the need to conduct an inquiry into homicides committed by someone who has been diagnosed with mental health problems. This has been criticised as further perpetuating a stereotype linking violence with mental illness. Taylor and Gunn (1999) analysed homicide statistics between 1957 and 1995 (during a growth in community care) and found that the rate of homicides committed by people with mental health problems remained stable while the overall murder rate rose. Marsden's (2006) analysis of homicides committed by people with severe mental illness showed that these accounted for less than half a per cent of all homicides in England and Wales. This is not to deny the tragedy that each one of these statistics represents. However, it is important to critically explore where the culture of risk assessment and management in mental health arises from.

It is within this context that Care Programme Approach policy was developed, the government announced a review of the Mental Health Act and risk assessment was incorporated into mental Care Programme Approach policy. This has been perceived as fulfilling an agenda to increase surveillance and monitoring in the community (Morrall & Muir-Cochrane 2002).

A number of authors also point to the changing nature of risk within wider society. Beck (1992) suggests that we now all live in a 'risk' society in which risks are global and as a society we become pre-occupied with achieving safety and managing risk. Lupton (1999) also highlights how the meaning of risk has changed from previously being associated with opportunity and chance to being dominated by a view of safety and control.

 Activity

> During your mental health placement, talk with a range of mental health professionals, exploring what their views are regarding risk assessment and management in mental health services. This may be developed into a question and answer discussion or reflective piece for your practice portfolio.

For some mental health professionals the dominance of risk and concern with a perceived link between violence and mental illness has contributed to a culture of blame in mental health services. Practitioners fear that the consequences of their actions may result in a tragic event for which they are held to blame. This can contribute to defensive practice in which decisions are made based upon this fear and an avoidance of situations where people may be exposed to being able to take chances. At best this can lead to hindering the recovery journey and at worst it can lead to unnecessary deprivation of liberty and compromise of personal autonomy. The following discussion explores effective risk assessment and management and considers how this can be conducted to attempt to avoid defensive practice.

Risks to people with mental health problems

It has been highlighted that risk of violence and risk of suicide are important areas for the assessment of risk. However, these are often focused on at the expense of other risks that service users are commonly exposed to. People with mental health problems are at greater risk of poverty and unemployment than other sectors of the population (Office of the Deputy Prime Minister 2004).

 Activity

> Identify a service user you have been working with on placement. Think about some of the risks that they have been exposed to during their use of services. You might want to think about the following:
>
> 1. Are they taking any medication? What are the short- or long-term side effects of this medication? (See the *British National Formulary* or BNF online for further information.)
> 2. What might be some of the potential risks of someone being in an in-patient environment with other people who are highly distressed?
> 3. What other treatments have they received which may have caused detrimental effects?
> 4. How have others responded to them as a result of their use of services? (Ch. 2 will provide some hints about the potential impact of this.)
>
> If you are working closely with an individual and have established a therapeutic relationship, these negative impacts of using services might be an issue that you want to talk through with them. This could also inform a reflective discussion.

There are potential risks posed in terms of social isolation, exploitation and risks posed by other service users and staff. Muir-Cochrane (2006) also examines the risk factors linked with developing physical health problems, particularly associated with schizophrenia. Chapter 2 highlighted that certain physical conditions are more common in people with mental health problems, representing increased risk to optimum physical health. There are also risks that are created by using mental health services; these are known as iatrogenic risks. The most common iatrogenic risks are the side effects and physical conditions, such as tardive dyskinesia, that may result from taking psychiatric medication. This highlights that the potential for risks associated with the experience of mental health problems are many and varied. It also recognises the need to examine the risks that the service user may be exposed to, which may fall outside the common factors highlighted in standardised risk assessment tools.

Risk assessment

Risk assessment has been defined as an examination of the context and the details of past risk incidents in the light of current circumstances. It entails the collection of information used to establish the likely occurrence of a future event and the impact and consequences of that event in terms of harms and benefits (Morgan 1998). In this respect there are two key aspects of the risk assessment process: identifying the potential consequences (the actions) and the potential likelihood of those consequences. It is important to bear in mind that risk can never be eliminated and it is very difficult to create accurate predictions for individuals (Royal College of Psychiatrists 2008). However, there is potential for practitioners and services to work in a way that helps to reduce the potential for risk.

There are two common types of risk assessment: actuarial and clinical. Actuarial approaches to risk assessment are based on statistical population information that is developed from research. They use this statistical information to make predictions in accordance with rules which are fixed (Buchanan 1999, Doyle & Dolan 2002). Risk assessment tools in mental health employ some actuarial measures. These include identifying issues such as unemployment and previous episodes of self-harm as risk factors for suicide, as population data suggest that these experiences are more common in people who have committed suicide.

Activity

Review the risk assessment tools that are used in your practice area. Can you identify any information in the assessments that you think may be based on an actuarial approach to risk assessment? The evidence base for different risk assessment tools is quite varied. However some, in particular those aiming to assess risk of violence, have been researched. Conduct a literature search to identify what evidence there is for the risk assessment tools used in your practice setting. This can support you with linking evidence and practice.

Clinical risk assessment refers to the more informal judgements that clinicians make. Assessment of risk is based on the clinician's understanding of the individual, their circumstances and relationships. The professional is able to respond flexibly to this understanding; for Doctor (2004) this involves engaging in the inner world of service users.

Risk assessment is a dynamic process which most commonly makes use of both clinical and actuarial approaches to inform judgements about the level and nature of risk. There are no risk assessment tools that have been standardised nationally though some have been validated through research. The Royal College of Psychiatrists (2008) has called for better evidence to support the development of tools to aid practitioners in the assessment of risk. It is therefore important to familiarise yourself with the risk assessment tools used within your clinical placement setting.

The usefulness of risk assessment for the mental health nurse is in its attempt to understand behaviour associated with risk. In this respect, risk assessment becomes an assessment of a current situation rather than an accurate predictor of a future event. Factors that may be taken into consideration in understanding behaviour associated with a risk include the following:

- Situational factors which may trigger or exacerbate risk behaviours.
- How key factors interact over time.
- The motivations behind behaviours.
- The consideration of context and environment.
- A need to include assessment of risks *to* the individual.

Developing this assessment helps to identify whether risks are high, medium or low and therefore informs the development of a risk management plan.

Case history

You arrive on shift and go around to say hello to the people on the ward. You find Zara in her room and she has a cut on each wrist. Zara was admitted last night and she is 20 years old. In handover you were told Zara has been displaying 'sexually disinhibited' behaviour. In the weeks before her admission she had been thrown out by her boyfriend and has been bunking in with friends since. Zara has been given a diagnosis of bipolar disorder. She had contact with adolescent services in the past. She has scars on her arm which you think might be from previous self-harm attempts. Zara's wounds are dressed and your mentor has spent some time talking with her. Your mentor asks you to help complete a risk assessment for Zara.

Reflection point

1. What potential risks are there for Zara?
2. What known risk factors are there for Zara?
3. What, if any, further information do you think you would need to complete a risk assessment?
4. What coping strategies, strengths and resources might Zara have based on the information given here?
5. Would you assess Zara as high, medium or low risk? In relation to what behaviour? What has informed your choice?

The learning and reflections you have conducted in this exercise could help you contribute to risk assessment in the practice setting. Discuss with your mentor the factors that you have identified here and how you may contribute to a risk assessment of someone you are working with in your placement area. Following this exercise, identify any further areas of learning you need in order to develop your skills in this area.

Risk management

Good quality risk assessment is important for managing risk (Royal College of Psychiatrists 2008). Risk management entails the development of plans that identify responsibilities and actions (Morgan 2000). These plans may be aiming to support, minimise or respond to behaviours associated with risk. Similar to any other plan within mental health services, there should be a date for review and evaluation of the plan. Risk management incorporates the decision-making process in which decisions are made based on knowledge of the evidence, of service users and their social context, of the service users' own experiences and the professionals' clinical judgement (DH 2007). This underpins the varied resources that are drawn upon in order to make decisions within health care and acknowledges that this is necessary to attempt to build an understanding of the complex factors that influence an individual's behaviour and use these to inform management. Risk is a changing concept and it is important to recognise that by helping to decrease some risks, others may increase. For example:

- Increasing medication dosage in an attempt to prevent a relapse may increase the risk of side effects from that medication.
- Placing someone on high observations may reduce the risk of self-harm but increase the risk that they may feel paranoid or disengage from working with practitioners.

Activity

Using the Case History on page 181 or using a risk assessment you have contributed to in your practice, consider:

1. Have there been any changes in the level of risk from when the assessment was previously completed?

2. If there have been changes, what has contributed to them? If there have been no changes, what has contributed to this?

Have a think about the different options for how the service might respond. You might want to think about the costs and benefits of each of these options. Remember, as a qualified professional you will not be making these decisions in isolation and would discuss them with the multidisciplinary team, service user and, where they are involved, their carers.

Multidisciplinary team working

Inquiries into homicides have consistently highlighted problems with communication within and across teams. Multidisciplinary team working enables the sharing of information and a more holistic picture of the situation to be established. It is also important to promote clarity within the planning process to help ensure each member is clear about their roles and responsibilities. It enables professionals to share expertise and can help challenge the culture of blame as decisions are made as a team. Developing risk assessment and management as a team also allows individual practitioners to listen to different perspectives and gain support for the challenges of working with risk in complex situations.

Collaboration with the service user

This involves considering the individual's perspective on their level of risk and the triggers and coping strategies in relation to this. Lagan and Lindow's (2004) research highlights that many service users want support to help minimise the potential for them to act in ways that might put others at risk.

Collaboration also creates space for service users to identify the areas that they feel pose a risk which may have been overlooked by professionals (such as the impact of medication or disempowerment through the mental health system) and ensures that plans also deal with these areas. Discussing potential risks needs to be sensitively handled and timing can be important. Collaboration is essential but collaborative risk assessment should be part of the therapeutic relationship to ensure that these issues can be discussed openly and people feel supported to address and develop responses to the identification of risks.

 Activity

Think about risk assessments that you have been involved in. If you are in the early stages of your course or you have not had the opportunity to contribute to a risk assessment, have a look at a risk assessment completed by a registered nurse. Explore how the service user has been involved in the risk assessment process. As the section above highlights, this can be a challenging and complex area to promote collaboration. This may also be an issue you want to discuss with your mentor.

Collaboration with family and carers where involved

Often those closest to the service user are able to observe most clearly the changes in that person's situation and behaviour. They are the people who tend to be the most likely victims of violent behaviour, should that arise. Marsden (2006) highlights that collaborating effectively with carers also involves reviewing management plans following the expression of concern on the part of carers and families. However, he also highlights how complex this issue can be. Within some families, antisocial behaviour is a norm and family situations can contribute to risk-associated actions. In relation to positive risk taking (see section below), families may find it difficult to support a service user to take chances for fear that their loved one may be being set up to fail and that they could be left to pick up the pieces.

Recognising individual strengths and resources

Working with individuals' strengths and resources within risk assessment is a central aspect of understanding risk (Royal College of Psychiatrists 2008). It is as important to explore the resources that help individuals cope with their distressing experiences and difficult circumstances as it is to identify the factors that are likely to trigger risks. This should help to support an individual's journey to recovery and promote greater understanding of the individual and their behaviour.

Positive risk taking

The central role that risk occupies within mental health practice coupled with the concerns regarding the potential for defensive practice have contributed to a call for a broader conceptualisation and approach to risk. Therapeutic or positive risk taking redefines risk to recognise the potential for benefits, opportunities and growth to occur as a result of taking a risk. Positive risk taking acknowledges that there are times when we should support people to take a risk in order to help them reach their goals and work towards recovery. Taking risks is what enables anyone to achieve in life and learn from their mistakes. Starting a new relationship, going for a job interview and taking a driving test all involve taking a risk which may succeed and pay off, but may also result in a loss from which we can often learn and develop ways of coping when supported with this process. Positive risk taking involves working with individuals to identify the courses of action they have available and supporting them to make decisions. In order to make choices, sharing information and examining the potential costs and benefits are important. Positive risk taking incorporates many choices an individual can make. Positive risk taking in practice might result in the following:

- Reducing or coming off psychiatric medication.
- Reducing levels of support.
- Starting a job.
- Moving to independent living following ongoing housing support.
- Taking a holiday.
- Developing a plan with someone around how to self-harm in the safest way possible.

Promoting positive risk taking involves many of the same approaches that contribute to effective risk assessment of known risks or perceived risk behaviours, such as therapeutic relationships with service users and their families, working as part of a team and developing relapse signatures and contingency plans. In addition, positive risk taking may be promoted through the following (Morgan 1998, 2000):

- Creative thinking.
- Exploring an individual's resources and past achievements.
- Working with service users to identify their limitations and abilities.
- Considering what resources are available in the community.
- Providing available and immediate support.
- Considering short-term increased risks in terms of long-term gains.

Positive risk taking has achieved support within more recent policy such as the ten essential shared capabilities (see Ch. 3) and the Department of Health's guide to best practice in risk assessment and management (DH 2007). These guidelines suggest that, in order to support positive risk taking, effective team working and clear documented plans are important (DH 2007). Team working and accessing supervision can be important for mental health nurses to gain support for enabling people to take therapeutic risks. An example can be seen in the following reflective learning exercise.

This chapter has provided an overview of risk assessment, management and therapeutic risk taking in contemporary mental health nursing practice. It has examined the significance of risk in relation to mental health services and suggested that this needs to be considered critically in relation to the social circumstances that have contributed to the situation. As mental health practitioners, it is important to situate an understanding of risk within the individual relationship that is developed with service users and to recognise the broader nature of risks that service users are exposed to.

Case history

Therapeutic risk taking

Mary wants to return to work; she tells you she is bored and would like something to do during the day. Mary is also building up debts and identifies work as a way of helping her with her finances. Mary continues to struggle with her obsessive thoughts which lead her to conduct cleaning rituals taking 90 minutes when she first gets up. Mary also has difficulties with her low mood and has a disturbed sleep pattern; she currently gets up at midday. You have been working with Mary on promoting healthy sleep and, during one-to-one sessions have developed a therapeutic relationship leading to Mary opening up about her obsessive thoughts. However, this has had limited impact on routines and waking time at this point. You explore the available options for work experience placements that would enable Mary to develop her CV, and have identified an opportunity to work in kennels which reflects her interests. However, you are concerned that she will not be able to arrive for the required start time.

Reflection point

1. What are your options for how you would proceed?
2. What course of action would support a positive risk taking approach?
3. What plans would you consider developing to support this course of action?
4. Reflecting on this exercise, what, if any, are your reservations about supporting positive risk taking? What do these represent?

Reflection point

Consider some of the service users you have been working with in practice. Can you identify any situations in which you think you and/or the team have taken positive risks with that person. In a reflective piece, consider what the impact of these positive risks was? What helped or hindered the process? How did you feel participating in this process?

References

Beck, U., 1992. Risk society: towards a new modernity. Sage, London.

Buchanan, A., 1999. Risk and dangerousness. Psychological Medicine 29, 465–473.

Department of Health, 1999. National service framework for mental health: modern standards and service models. HMSO, London.

Department of Health, 2004. Essential shared capabilities: a framework for the whole of the mental health workforce. HMSO, London.

Department of Health, 2006. From values to action: the Chief Nursing Officer's review of mental health nursing. HMSO, London.

Department of Health, 2007. Best practice in managing risk: principles and evidence for best practice in the assessment and management of risk to self and others in mental health services. HMSO, London.

Doctor, R., 2004. Psychodynamic lessons in risk assessment and management. Advances in Psychiatric Treatment 10, 267–276.

Doyle, M., Dolan, M., 2002. Violence risk assessment: combining actuarial and clinical information to structure clinical judgements for the formulation and management of risk. Journal of Psychiatric and Mental Health Nursing 9 (6), 649–657.

Lagan, J., Lindow, V., 2004. Living with risk: mental health service user involvement in risk assessment and management. Policy Press, Bristol.

Lupton, D., 1999. Risk (key ideas). Routledge, London.

Marsden, T., 2006. Review of homicides by patients with severe mental illness. Imperial College, London.

Morgan, S., 1998. Assessing and managing risk: a training pack for practitioners and managers of comprehensive mental health services. Pavilion, Brighton.

Morgan, S., 2000. Clinical risk management: a clinical tool and practitioner manual. The Sainsbury Centre for Mental Health, London.

Morrall, P., Muir-Cochrane, E., 2002. Naked social control: seclusion and psychiatric nursing in post-liberal society. Australian e-journal for the Advancement of Mental Health 1 (2), 2–12.

Muir-Cochrane, E., 2006. Medical co-morbidity risk factors and barriers to care for people with schizophrenia. Journal of Psychiatric and Mental Health Nursing 13, 447–452.

Office of the Deputy Prime Minister, 2004. Social exclusion unit report. ODPM, London.

Paterson, B., Stark, 2001. Social policy and mental illness in England in the 1990s: violence, moral panic and critical discourse. Journal of Psychiatric and Mental Health Nursing 8, 257–267.

Repper, J., Perkins, R., 2003. Social inclusion and recovery. Baillière Tindall, Edinburgh.

Royal College of Psychiatrists, 2008. Rethinking risk to others in mental health services. Royal College of Psychiatrists, London.

Taylor, P., Gunn, J., 1999. Homicides by people with mental illness; myth and reality. British Journal of Psychiatry 174 (9), 14.

Further reading

Department of Health, 2007. Best practice in managing risk: principles and evidence for best practice in the assessment and management of risk to self and others in mental health services. HMSO, London.

Felton, A., Bertram, G., 2008. Positive risk taking: a framework for practice. In: Stickley, T., Bassett, T. (Eds.), Learning about mental health practice. Wiley, Chichester.

Lagan, J., Lindow, V., 2004. Living with risk: mental health service user involvement in risk assessment and management. Policy Press, Bristol.

Websites

Website produced by Steve Morgan who has developed a number of resources for positive risk taking, http://practicebasedevidence.squarespace.com (accessed June 2011).

13 Handling difficult situations

Victoria Baldwin

CHAPTER AIMS

- To develop an understanding of different types of behaviour and what factors may impact on how service users behave and interact
- To reflect on the impact of difficult interactions on you as a student nurse, and how to manage this within your practice
- To explore a range of therapeutic skills which can be used in a range of difficult interactions to support you in meeting the service user's needs
- To identify different interactions which can be perceived as difficult and explore specific strategies to support you in responding effectively

Introduction

As a student mental health nurse on placement, there will be times when you will come across what will be referred to in this chapter as 'difficult situations'. These situations may involve a number of experiences related to working in mental health, including responding to self-harm,

suicidal thoughts or managing aggressive or distressing behaviour. However, these difficult situations may also be times when you work with service users who, due to their complex experiences, feel very difficult to understand and engage with, for example working with service users given a diagnosis of personality disorder. The emotional response we have as a student mental health nurse impacts on how able we feel to cope and respond effectively to difficult situations.

This chapter will explore some of these situations and consider different approaches to understanding these experiences to allow you as a student nurse to react in a way that is safe and engaging. A number of scenarios and examples will be highlighted which you may encounter on your placements to help you explore different ways of responding within these difficult situations, and also support you in developing confidence to manage difficult or challenging service users.

The impact of past experience on current behaviour

An important aspect when exploring how service users behave is their early life and developmental experiences and how some of these experiences may be influencing their reactions and responses in the present. Young et al (2003) identify a number of core emotional needs to support the development of children into healthy adults. These core emotional needs include aspects such as:

- forming secure attachments to others
- having the freedom to express valid needs and emotions
- having the opportunity to act spontaneously and exercise self-control.

Throughout our early development it is important that these core emotional needs are met through either our parents or care providers. If these core emotional needs are not met, it may have an impact on how we view ourselves as an adult and how we view others and the world around us. The influence of early life experiences is particularly relevant for service users who may have experienced neglect, trauma or abuse within their early development and, as a result, may have difficulties relating to people within a position of providing care. As a mental health nurse, we may expect service users to perceive us positively. However, if a service user has grown up in an environment where their provider of care has been neglectful or abusive, they may develop an expectation that you as a nurse may be abusive or neglectful. If a service user has been abandoned as a child or experienced inconsistent parenting, then they may perceive you as being potentially abandoning or may expect you to reject them or provide inconsistent support. In light of this, they may be cautious of forming an engaging relationship with you. In order to address this, it is important to constantly reinforce your commitment to support the development of a healthy working relationship with the service user and remain consistent in your approach to reinforcing this message.

Managing and making sense of difficult situations

When faced with difficult or challenging situations, it is important that you are able to think about and reflect on what the service user is communicating alongside managing your own responses. This will enable you to support the service user with their individual needs and manage the situation effectively. In order to do this, a simple framework can be used which involves three key stages. First, it is important to try and make sense of what the service user is feeling. Second, it is important to be mindful and aware of your own feelings and then, by using both perspectives, the final stage involves exploring how to respond effectively. These stages are explored below in more detail using examples to demonstrate key points.

What is the service user feeling?

It is important when understanding behaviour to think about how the service user might actually be feeling. This can be viewed as an assessment process providing an opportunity to think about what specific factors may be influencing feelings and how this links to current behaviour. Key aspects to be aware of when exploring how a service user is feeling may include the following:

The service user's experience of services, both past and present This is important to allow you as a student nurse to create a picture of what the service user's expectations of you may be.

The service user's early developmental experiences and past experiences of relationships This may provide you with more information about how the service user reacts to specific situations and how they might perceive caring services.

The aspirations and goals of the service user and what they hope to achieve from the therapeutic relationship This will help you to understand how the service user may perceive the relationship and what aspects they may find challenging.

Individual triggers Individual triggers can be generated in collaboration with service users following specific interactions or periods of crisis, whereby the service user highlights areas of difficulty which may invoke strong emotions or reactions, or cause a challenge.

How am I feeling?

When working with service users that present with difficult behaviour, it can cause a range of feelings and emotions and we can feel challenged on an individual level, both personally and professionally. The emphasis is often placed solely on how we respond to the service user rather than exploring what you as a student nurse might be feeling and the impact of this. If you are aware that a difficult interaction has made you feel anxious or scared, it is important to think about how this might influence your ability to provide support in an authentic way. Alternatively, if an interaction has made you feel frustrated or disappointed, it is likely that this may be evident in how you respond if you have not made sense of this and managed your response.

An interesting element of exploring both your own and the service user's feelings is that there is often a parallel between these feelings. For example, when a service user is aggressive, they may be feeling anxious and scared and, as a result, you may also start to feel anxious and scared. By exploring both sets of feelings and experiences together, you may identify specific factors that have impacted on the interaction and create a more in-depth understanding of what has happened within the interaction.

You may be surprised by your reaction to some behaviours. This may be because a situation reminds you of a past personal or professional experience and evokes emotions

which you were not aware were still present. You may also question if the way you are feeling is 'appropriate' in light of your role and the expectations you have placed upon yourself or the expectations you perceive others have of you. Many students describe feeling guilty that they didn't know how to respond to a difficult situation, unprofessional because they wanted to cry in response to an upsetting experience or cowardly because they felt scared by a service user's aggression. All too often these feelings are hidden and can result in negative ways of coping such as avoiding a service user, referring to them in a derogatory way or allowing the feelings to transfer to other aspects of life. The ability to recognise and acknowledge this requires a high level of self-awareness and can be processed safely in a clinical supervision setting or through personal reflection.

How to respond effectively

Once you have made sense of a difficult interaction, you will then be in a position to use this information to think about how to respond effectively. It is important to remember to see the behaviour or difficulty as a communication of an unmet need and respond to this rather than place judgement on the service user.

Specific skills in responding effectively

When working with difficult interactions, there are a number of skills that can be applied to help you respond effectively. The following framework identifies these skills, and you will notice that a number of them are expanded upon in previous sections of this book.

Effective communication

It is important to think about effective verbal communication such as tone of voice, pace and demonstrating active listening. During times of distress or frustration, be mindful of how you may project some of these feelings through your non-verbal communication such as body language.

Maintaining a positive approach to engagement

Whether you are supporting a service user experiencing high levels of distress or someone who is responding aggressively towards you, it is important to maintain a positive approach to engagement. Service users who present with difficult behaviours may evoke strong negative responses in you or your peers, and at times it can be hard to manage these responses which can result in a negative or, in some cases, punitive response towards the service user.

Validation

The main purpose of validation is to demonstrate that you recognise that the service user is experiencing high levels of distress and that, although your role as a worker is to try and alleviate this distress, you are not in any way minimising the effect of this distress or the nature of it.

Example You are on placement in a community mental health team and have been working with a service user who has a diagnosis of anxiety and depression. When you attend on your next visit, she presents to you as extremely distressed about a break up in a relationship. You are aware from discussing this service user with your mentor that this has happened previously and that the relationship has been unstable for some time. It is more important to validate her experience by acknowledging the level of distress the break up may cause and to offer support in response to this. Once you have validated her distress, it may then be appropriate to encourage her to reflect on what skills or strategies she has used previously to manage this distress.

Demonstrating collaborative working

It is important to constantly be mindful of the collaborative nature of the therapeutic relationship and, even during times of distress, it is important to involve the service users in decisions that are made and management plans that are put in place.

Being clear about what support is available

When working with service users, it is important to be very clear at the outset about how much support and time are available from you within your role, and to identify access to further support when required, such as out-of-hours support. As you may only be on placement for a short time, it may be helpful to highlight this with service users so that they are clear from the start about the limits of your ongoing involvement in their care.

Consistency

By maintaining consistency, you will also help service users to know what support is available and in what circumstances they are able to access support. It is important to acknowledge that it is likely that service users will have experienced inconsistent support and engagement from some staff or services. This can be challenging for service users and may create more feelings of distress if they are unsure if support is available. It is your responsibility to be clear about the working relationship from the first interaction and maintain this consistency throughout your work as best as possible within the limits of the time you have available on your placements.

Self-awareness

It is important to constantly be aware of your own feelings and experiences within the therapeutic relationship. As we have explored earlier, when working with difficult situations your feelings will often parallel those of the service user, however it is important that you are aware of this and manage it effectively to enable you to support the service user with their experiences and emotions. It may be helpful to use a reflective model (such as Gibbs' (1988) reflective cycle or Rolfe's framework for reflective practice (Rolfe et al 2001)) during supervision or reflective practice to enable you to develop your self-awareness and manage your own feelings effectively. It may be helpful to explore this with your mentor when discussing your progress on your placements.

Providing a feeling of safety for the service user through containment

When working with service users, it is important as a student nurse to provide a feeling of safety to support them with their difficult experiences. This has been referred to as offering containment or containing a person's feelings. In Bion's (1962) early work, the concept was referred to as a mechanism for managing distressing or unmanageable feelings. The container is referred to as a space to take unmanageable emotions and experiences and transfer them into something manageable. In the context of working with service users, the container is the relationship between you as the student nurse and the service user. Service users who may be extremely distressed or experiencing difficult symptoms may not be able to make sense of their experiences due to the unmanageable nature of them. By offering support and helping the service user make sense of these difficult experiences, you are containing their distress.

Maintaining boundaries

It is important for you as a student nurse to be very clear about the boundaries of a relationship and ensure the service user is aware of these boundaries. The term 'boundary' has been referred to as a therapeutic frame which defines the characteristics of the therapeutic relationship (Gutheil & Gabbard 1993). However, in mental health, assumptions are made regarding boundaries and who asserts them and there is often a lack of clarity about what these boundaries are and who defines them. When boundaries are 'crossed' or 'broken', the blame can often fall on the

service user who has been perceived to 'push the boundary' or 'cross the boundary'. However, often service users are not aware of the boundaries in place, and therefore may struggle to understand the consequences of when boundaries are broken. It is unfair to expect service users to maintain therapeutic boundaries in the relationship without being involved in any discussion regarding these boundaries. Therefore, it is important to be clear about the boundaries of engagement with service users at the start of a relationship and continue to explore these with the service user throughout the period of the relationship.

Examples Claire is 28 years old and has a diagnosis of borderline personality disorder and was recently discharged from an acute ward where you are currently on placement. Claire contacts the acute ward by telephone within the last 10 minutes of your shift and asks for some support. Initially you are unsure as you are aware your shift is due to finish, however you feel you need to offer Claire support to ensure she is OK before you leave. Rather than offer unlimited support, you explain to Claire that, although you are concerned about her distress, you are due to finish your shift shortly. You identify that you can offer 5 minutes now before you leave and, alongside that, you can either identify who is available on the next shift to give support or arrange a time when you are next on shift to offer further support. By approaching the situation in this way, you have validated Claire's distress, reinforced the boundary of how much support you can offer and also provided alternative suggestions for accessing support if Claire requires this.

Responding effectively to specific difficult situations

Having explored some of the interventions and approaches that can support you to manage difficult interactions that you might experience with a service user, the following section of this chapter will highlight specific issues in relation to a number of interactions commonly experienced with mental health service users. Remember to refer back to the previous section and explore how these skills can be used in all your interactions with service users.

Making sense of, and responding positively to, anger or aggression

Working with service users who display aggressive behaviours can be extremely challenging for student nurses and can cause you to experience a range of emotions. In order to work effectively with service users, it is important to see this form of behaviour as any other form and try to read what the service user is trying to communicate. Quirk et al (2004) identify that service users take an active role in making a safe environment for themselves and are not passive recipients of care. This is a result of feeling unable to rely on staff to ensure their safety. In light of this, service users may be aware of how to keep themselves safe during difficult times and it is important to engage them in this process. Carlsson et al (2000) have identified a number of themes in supporting the management of aggression including respecting your own fear and respecting the service user. They also highlight the importance of providing stability for the service user during times of distress and aggression.

A number of the skills previously discussed may be helpful in managing these interactions and experiences, for example effective communication and validation. However, there are also a number of specific issues to be aware of when responding effectively to service users who appear angry or aggressive:

- Try to use your understanding of the framework discussed earlier to think about what the service user might be feeling and what messages are being communicated. It is also helpful to think about other factors that might be

impacting on the interaction such as the environment, other service users and previous experiences.
- It is always important to remain calm in your own posture and position within the environment and try to respond positively. Try to maintain a supportive but non-confrontational posture.
- Show your concern and use validation to empathise with the service user before trying to manage the situation. By doing this you are acknowledging that the service user is trying to communicate a difficult experience and you are demonstrating that you are willing to work with the them to help with this experience rather than make a quick judgement about their response.
- Try to guide the service user to a place of safety within the environment where it may be appropriate to spend time and offer support.
- Be mindful of your non-verbal communication and how this may be perceived by the service user.
- Once the service user has accessed support and appears calmer, it may be helpful to explore with them the cause of the aggression by encouraging them to reflect on what factors may have impacted on their behaviour.

> ✅ **Tip**
>
> As a nurse, your role is to support the service user to make sense of their experiences. Therefore, following a difficult interaction, once this has been resolved and the service user has accessed support, it is important that you explore with the service user what happened and help them to make sense of why they responded in the way they did. By doing this, you are helping the service user to use the framework in a helpful way which may support them in their recovery process.

Case history

Susan is 37 years old and has been in contact with services for a number of years, both as an in-patient and in community services. Susan has recently been readmitted to an in-patient ward and is approached by one of the staff nurses on shift to try and complete an assessment. In response to questions asked by the nurse, Susan becomes aggressive and starts shouting at the nurse: "What's the point in answering these f**king questions when you are only going to try and get rid of me as soon as possible?"

Reflection point

Use the framework discussed above to explore what is happening within this situation. What factors might be influencing this interaction?

Possible ways of responding:

■ Validate Susan's distress by acknowledging that the assessment process can be frustrating or appear intimidating.

■ Reinforce your commitment to offer support in helping Susan with this process by offering to work through the assessment with her.

■ Encourage Susan to move to a quiet area away from other service users on the ward so you will be able to offer support.

■ Suggest you complete part of the assessment together now and negotiate another time to complete the assessment when Susan feels more comfortable.

Working effectively with self-harm

Working with service users who self-harm can be a complex process and, as a student nurse, there may be times when you feel overwhelmed by the responsibility of managing this type of risk. However, it is important to try and remember that the same principles of engagement apply when working with self-harm, and the skills we discussed previously can help you in working with such service users. It is also important to work collaboratively with your mentor to explore how to work positively with different types of risk in a safe and contained way.

Motz (2009) highlights the importance of understanding self-harm as a form of communication which requires an urgent response. Self-harm is a way of coping with the extreme levels of distress an individual may be coping with. It may also be a result of the service user being unable to regulate their emotions in such a way as to manage the unbearable feelings they are

experiencing. Motz (2009) identifies that, although the process of self-harm can be perceived as negative, the message behind it can often be of hope and a will to stay alive. A number of studies have been completed exploring the views of service users who self-harm and the results indicate that, in all circumstances, people need an empathic non-judgemental approach to their self-harming behaviour. This should be based on practitioners having an understanding of the issues involved alongside the functions self-harm may fulfil for that individual (Royal College of Psychiatrists 2010). In light of this, the first key aim of engagement is to respond in a way that validates the experience of the service user and carries no judgement regarding your views regarding self-harm.

Key issues to remember

- Collaborative assessment to explore the service user's experiences and feelings is essential and will act as a basis for any further support and intervention. A biopsychosocial assessment is recommended to be completed by an experienced practitioner as highlighted within the National Institute for Health and Clinical Excellence (NICE) guidelines (2004). Assessment should seek to identify developmental aspects that may highlight particular experiences the service user is struggling with and other mental health symptoms or experiences. Particular triggers or precipitating factors during times of high distress should also be explored to try and develop support mechanisms where appropriate. As a student nurse, you may be in a position to support this assessment process, but should seek support from a more experienced nurse to complete the full assessment.

- Develop a care plan with the service user highlighting specific triggers and factors that might precipitate self-harm and helpful coping strategies that can be implemented to minimise harm.
- In response to assessment, the service user should be provided with appropriate support, both directly linked to the physical self-harm in terms of pain minimisation and also support with the specific areas of distress highlighted during the assessment process.
- It is important to access support and supervision to help make sense of some of your emotions associated with working with service users who self-harm. This will enable you to support the service user effectively by managing your own experiences.
- Inspiring hope within the service user is increasingly important when working in mental health and with service users who self-harm. It is your responsibility as a student nurse to nurture hope and, even in times of uncertainty, to retain this and model this for the service user.
- Although we have highlighted that self-harm and suicide are different, it is

important to remember that self-harm is a risk factor for suicide and research has suggested that 30–40% of people who have died by suicide have self-harmed within the previous 2 years (Gunnell et al 2005). Therefore, when working with service users who self-harm, assessment for risk of suicide should always take place.

Further support and guidance on working with service users who self-harm can be accessed by the NICE guidelines for self-harm (2004).

Working effectively with service users expressing suicidal thoughts

Although self-harm and suicide have often been referred to in the same light, it is also important to acknowledge that they are very different and, though they clearly have links, should be managed as separate issues and may require different approaches. As previously identified, self-harm is a risk factor for suicide, and assessment is fundamental in ascertaining the underlying factors that may be causing the service user to feel such high levels of distress or hopelessness. However, Szmukler (2003) highlights the complexity of assessing suicide risk accurately and, in light of this, emphasises the importance of psychosocial assessments completed through engaging with the service user on an individual level and hearing their experiences rather than relying on complex tools.

Furthermore, Burke et al (2008) highlight that what is most helpful in working with service users is the development of a relationship in which they are listened to and supported and that judgements are not made regarding the intent for suicide. Further, he suggests that ensuring boundaries are clear about the relationship can provide a framework for support. Other areas to be aware of when working with service users are highlighted include the following:

- Expression of suicidal thoughts should always be taken seriously, even if you have worked with a service user on another placement and have seen similar expressions that have not been acted on.
- Assessment of suicide risk is important and should be an ongoing collaborative process when working with service users expressing suicidal thoughts. Refer to Chapter 12 on assessing and managing risk to ensure an appropriate risk assessment has taken place and all factors that may indicate suicide risk have been explored.
- Access support from your mentor to ensure you feel able to manage interactions with the service user. It is important to work collaboratively within the wider team to ensure a consistent approach to responding to these issues and to ensure you are aware of any care plans that are in place to respond to increasing levels of risk. Effective communication and documentation to ensure all areas have been considered is imperative to maintain the safety of the service user, yourself and the wider team.
- Try to engage the service user and ensure the therapeutic relationship is maintained to provide an open forum to explore some of these issues in a meaningful way.
- Don't be afraid to explore the issues with the service user as this will demonstrate to the service user you are aware of their experiences and you are available for support. It may be helpful to support the service user in identifying potential triggers increasing their distressing thoughts and also protective factors that may manage difficult feelings.
- When working in the community, referral to the crisis or out-of-hours service may be needed to ensure the service user has access to support if you have concerns about their safety outside of your placement hours.

- Access supervision and support from your mentor or link tutor to help you manage difficult interactions or feelings associated with service users who express suicidal thoughts.

Knowing when to engage further support or services

Although there are a number of skills that can be helpful in working with service users during difficult interactions, there will be times when the skills you have developed or the interventions you have implemented may not be helpful or may not be enough to support a service user in times of distress. In light of this, you may need to explore support from your mentor, other staff members working in your placement area or other services to ensure the service user and you remain safe and that the service user has access to the required support. Knowing when to access further support or engage other services is an important skill for a developing nurse and should not be underestimated. If you are working with a service user and have concerns regarding your ability to provide enough support or how effective your approach is, it may be helpful to consider one or more of the following options:

- Seek guidance and support from your mentor or a more experienced member of the team regarding your approach. This could be approached on an individual level or through a forum such as handover or group supervision.
- Explore opportunities for further input within the team in terms of specific therapeutic interventions or approaches. There may be a member of the team who has worked with service users experiencing similar difficulties before who may be able to offer support and guidance.
- Co-work with or shadow a more experienced member of the team to

provide support and guidance when working with a service user that you are finding difficult.

- If you have concerns about the safety of a service user outside of your placement hours, there may be the opportunity to refer the service user to a crisis team or relevant out-of-hours service.
- Refer to specialist services if a clear rationale is available and inclusion criteria are appropriate for the specified service.

References

Bion, S., 1962. Learning from experience. Heinemann, London.

Burke, M., Duffy, D., Trainor, G., et al., 2008. Self-injury – a recovery and evidence based toolkit. Salford and Trafford Mental Health NHS Trust, Bolton.

Carlsson, G., Dahlberg, K., Drew, N., 2000. Encountering violence and aggression in mental health nursing: a phenomenological study of tacit caring knowledge. Issues in Mental Health Nursing 21, 533–545.

Gibbs, G., 1988. Learning by doing: a guide to teaching and learning methods. Further Education Unit, Oxford Polytechnic, Oxford.

Gunnell, D., Bennewith, O., Peters, T., et al., 2005. The epidemiology and management of self-harm amongst adults in England. Journal of Public Health (Bangkok) 27 (1), 67–73.

Gutheil, T.G., Gabbard, G.O., 1993. The concept of boundaries in clinical practice: theoretical and risk-management dimensions. American Journal of Psychiatry 150, 188–196.

Motz, A., 2009. Managing self harm: psychological perspectives. Routledge, Sussex.

National Institute for Health and Clinical Excellence, 2004. The short-term physical and psychological management and secondary prevention of self-harm in primary and secondary care. NICE, London.

Quirk, A., Lelliott, P., Seale, C., 2004. Service users' strategies for managing risk in the volatile environment of an acute psychiatric ward. Social Science and Medicine 59 (12), 2573–2583.

Rolfe, G., Freshwater, D., Jasper, M., 2001. Critical reflection for nursing and the helping professions. Palgrave, Basingstoke.

Royal College of Psychiatrists, 2010. Self-harm, suicide and risk: helping people who self-harm. Royal College of Psychiatrists College Report, London.

Szmukler, G., 2003. Risk assessment: 'numbers' and 'values'. Psychiatric Bulletin 27, 205–207.

Young, J.E., Klosko, J.S., Weishaar, M.E., 2003. Schema therapy: a practitioner's guide. Guilford, New York.

Further reading

Aieyegbusi, A., 2004. Thinking under fire: the challenge for forensic mental health nurses working with women in secure care. In: Jeffcote, N., Watson, T. (Eds.), Working therapeutically with women in secure settings. Jessica Kingsley, London.

National Institute for Health and Clinical Excellence, 2004. New guidelines for standardising care for people who self-harm. NICE, London.

National Institute for Health and Clinical Excellence, 2009. Borderline personality disorder: the NICE guidelines on treatment and management. NICE, London.

Websites

Service users' personal accounts of self-harm-http://www.mind.org.uk.

A psychiatrist's experience of assessing risk-http://www.patientvoices.org.uk/flv/0441pv384.htm.

14 Demonstrating leadership in a mental health setting

CHAPTER AIMS

- To gain an insight into leadership within nursing and clinical practice
- To outline mental health practice examples where leadership may be demonstrated
- To understand the case management approach
- To examine working in partnership with different organisations

Introduction

This chapter looks at the issue of leadership in nursing practice and applies this to mental health settings through reflective learning exercises. In doing so, it considers the importance of leading care through commonly used approaches in mental health settings such as case management. Leadership, case management and partnership working are domains of competence in the Nursing and Midwifery Council (NMC) standards (NMC 2008).

Leadership

A good leader is one who is able to make things happen, to provide inspiration to others to innovate and develop practice (Williamson et al 2008). Delivering good quality care within mental health nursing involves being an effective leader. This section explores what leadership in nursing care is, examines the skills that this involves and considers some situations where you might demonstrate leadership.

Leadership in nursing can be examined from a number of perspectives. First, as Williamson et al (2008) demonstrate, it may be considered for its central role in developing and delivering quality health care and impacting positively on the lives of individuals and families who use services. Lord Darzi (Department of Health (DH) 2008) highlights that strong clinical leadership is the bedrock of empowering both staff and patients in the NHS to ensure high standards of clinical care. In this respect, leadership relates to the development of nursing practice. Kitson (2001) suggests that leadership is about making visions into reality. However, Antrobus and Kitson (1999) highlight that leadership in nursing is also about influencing the health policy that shapes the way in which health care is delivered. This involves developing nursing knowledge and influencing others at a different level, through involvement in regional and national forums, management and research. All forms of leadership involve providing a role model and support to others which helps to promote good nursing care (DH 2006a). The Chief Nursing Officer's review of mental health nursing (DH 2006b) points out that leaders are to be found at every level of an organisation.

 Reflection point

Think of someone who you would define as a good leader. This could be someone you have worked with in mental health practice, in previous jobs or a peer. What is it that makes them a good leader? Make a list of what skills, qualities and attributes are important.

Identify how you might be able to incorporate some of these skills/ attributes into the delivery of care.

It is common for people to confuse leadership and management. While they share some roles and key skills, this confusion is based on a misunderstanding of the terms and has the potential to inhibit the development of effective leadership in nursing practice. Delivering good quality nursing care involves leadership. Of course those who manage will also be required to be leaders and vice versa, yet it is important that we don't see leadership as a hierarchical concept which is only the remit of those in senior positions in health care.

There is a wealth of literature that examines the similarities and differences between leadership and management. Kotter (1990a,b) highlights that a manager's key role is in dealing with complexity while a leader's role is in creating change (Table 14.1).

As a student mental health nurse, particularly during the latter part of your

Table 14.1 Leadership and management

Leaders	Managers
Define direction	Organise resources and plan
Bring people together	
Inspire and motivate others	Organise staff
	Control problems

(Ramsden 1998)

course, there may be a number of activities you are involved in that entail adopting the role of leader.

Activity

Make a list of the activities that you have been involved in, in mental health practice where you have shown leadership skills or acted as a leader. It may help you to think about what worked well in these situations and what didn't work so well. This can be used as the basis for a reflective piece or to develop an action plan for continuing to build on your leadership skills. It may also be helpful to revisit what you have produced in this exercise when completing job applications to help you highlight this skill and how you have used it on your practice placement.

Outlined below are a few examples of such areas and a breakdown of the skills and approaches that may assist you in developing leadership in these areas.

Chairing a care programme approach review
• Good time keeping:
  – agreeing start and finish times
  – periodically reminding people of the time left available
  – if necessary, asking people to move on to the next point.

- Making people feel welcome:
  - thinking about the environment
  - is the room set up to facilitate communication?
  - offering refreshments.
- Facilitating the meeting:
  - allowing everyone to have a say
  - opening and ending the meeting
  - summarising what has been decided.

Coordinating a shift

- Clarifying tasks and requirements:
  - recognising what needs to be done and when
  - recognising and communicating what may not be possible.
- Effectively managing resources:
  - identifying what resources you have available
  - taking into consideration resources such as time, people and space.
- Delegation:
  - considering who is best placed to complete a task
  - might include considering team members' skills, relationships, resources and limitations
  - checking out delegated tasks have been completed
  - offering support
  - providing clear instruction
  - trusting others
  - recognising that to be effective you can't do everything yourself!
- Communication:
  - keeping people (staff and people using the service) informed of what's going on
  - documenting decisions and the rationale
  - recording relevant information in required records
  - handing over information.
- Keeping calm:
  - there are no easy answers for this one but it is essential to take time if needed to think things over and to take your breaks.

Key working (or co-key working)

- Developing trust:
  - using interpersonal skills effectively to establish therapeutic relationships
  - exploring strengths, wishes and goals alongside problems and needs.
- Prioritising support/interventions:
  - collaboratively making decisions about care
  - developing plans of care
  - evaluating progress and plans in light of changes.
- Effective team working:
  - identifying and valuing the contribution of others to an individual's care
  - communicating what is being done and by who to reduce duplication of work and confusion
  - this may include contacting and involving family and friends as requested by the individual.
- Delegation:
  - breaking down steps required to work towards care plan aims and identifying who will support the service user to achieve these aims
  - setting timelines for achievement.
- Ending:
  - planning for the end of therapeutic relationships (see Ch. 7)
  - identifying and planning for how the work you have been doing will be continued after placement.

Facilitating multidisciplinary meetings

This may share some skills with chairing a Care Programme Approach (CPA) review such as good organisational and time management skills. However, there are a few additional areas to consider:

- Advocacy:
  - service users are still quite invisible in multidisciplinary team decision making, therefore you may be required to represent the views of an individual you are working with
  - this could include asserting the case for the course of action they prefer.

- Containment:
  - discussion may involve debating a number of different perspectives; as a facilitator, there is a role in inviting people to speak to ensure every voice is heard and perhaps asking others to listen
  - summarising the discussion and the decision reached and acknowledging differences is important.
- Feedback and follow up:
  - agreeing what action needs to be taken
  - feeding this back to the rest of the team or agreeing the means through which this will be communicated (e.g. amendment to a care plan, running records, handover)
  - agreeing the means through which this will be reviewed and evaluated (e.g. does this need to be discussed at the next meeting?).

This has provided a brief outline of some activities where as a nursing student or practitioner you may be acting as a leader. The breakdown of these areas provides some insight into the complexity of leadership in clinical care. This list is far from extensive but your involvement in such areas will help you work towards achieving your NMC competencies. The following section considers an example from mental health nursing practice where you may be asked to demonstrate leadership, both as a student and qualified practitioner, and asks you to think about some of the implications of what this involves. It is possible that you have already encountered situations which raise similar issues in your own practice. It may help to think about these in the context of the following scenarios and examine whether you would take a similar course of action again and if your experiences on your course have influenced this at all.

Scenario

Jodie is the deputy team leader on Partridge Unit. She is an experienced professional and your associate mentor. It is 10.00 a.m. and

Jodie asks you to accompany her to go around the unit to let the people know that the anxiety management group is about to start. Jodie goes around every room and walks straight in without knocking.

1. What, if any, are your concerns in relation to this scenario?
2. How might the people on the unit feel about Jodie's approach?

Jodie walks into Abhid's room and wakes him up. Abhid returned to the unit at 2.00 a.m. and had disturbed sleep. Abhid shouts at Jodie and becomes angry. Jodie states she is not interested, slams the door and continues around. Jodie walks straight in to Roy's room. He has just returned from the shower and is undressed. Jodie returns to the office and tells Kirsty, a healthcare assistant new to the unit. They giggle about Abhid's reaction and Roy's state of undress.

1. What principle is Jodie disrespecting?
2. What policy and evidence is there that challenges Jodies approach?

You are deeply concerned about Jodie's behaviour. How do you react? Think about this for a moment and then pick one of the options below which most closely represents the course of action that you might take.

A. Ignore your feelings of discomfort and don't say anything.
B. Interrupt Kirsty and Jodie and say you are disgusted with what Jodie did and feel that their behaviour is completely inappropriate.
C. Tell the staff that you have befriended on the unit that you think Jodie was out of order and she doesn't know what she is doing.
D. Discuss your concerns with your mentor and ask them to have a word.
E. Discuss your concerns with your mentor, then meet with Jodie to share how you felt about how she behaved.

Option A

This may well be a common reaction. The scenario identified Jodie as a senior clinician in the team. Some students may not trust their reactions or knowledge of the situation. There may also be a fear that if you were to say anything to Jodie, this could impact on your own assessment and feedback. However, it is possible that not dealing with such feelings of discomfort and ignoring the impact they may have could contribute to the stress and perceived emotional costs of nursing. According to the NMC code, a nurse must act to promote dignity at all times and that poor care is not acceptable (NMC 2008).

Option B

This acknowledges the previous point in terms of highlighting that poor care is unacceptable. However, communicating concerns to Jodie in this manner appears confrontational and has the potential to be shared in an aggressive rather than assertive manner.

Option C

Again this option highlights that you have identified a concern with the manner in which Jodie practised in this particular situation and this may be interpreted as a means for you to access support from other people. Effective team working is supported by open communication and honesty, and reacting in this way has the potential to impact negatively on team working as resentment may build towards Jodie. It also doesn't necessarily provide a good role model for the remainder of the team.

Option D

The literature consistently links quality leadership with both the provision of support but also the need for people who are leaders to be supported (DH 2006a, 2008). This option allows you to raise your concerns about the quality of care being delivered and also gain support. This may be the most appropriate option depending on the context in which poor practice is observed and your own confidence and development.

Option E

Through sharing your views with your mentor, you are able to check out the concerns identified in option A in terms of your own understanding, knowledge and reaction to the situation. This also reflects the requirements of your competencies to participate in supervision and reflect on how your values and emotions impact on your leadership practice. However, leadership is also about maintaining standards and striving for quality. Through addressing your concerns directly with Jodie appropriately and professionally, you are also acting as an advocate for the service users and families who may be under your care. Chapter 13 includes a section on assertiveness. However, these are some suggestions for how the concerns may be broached with Jodie:

1. At the School of Nursing, we recently talked a lot about privacy and I read about essence of care. In relation to this, I was feeling a bit concerned when we didn't knock on Abhid's and Roy's doors to let them know about the anxiety group. Do you think it would have been better if we had asked before going into their rooms?

2. Thank you for your help on Tuesday and I enjoyed getting involved in the preparation for the anxiety group. However, I have not seen Abhid angry before and am a bit worried that us going straight into his room may have upset him. What do you think about how the situation was approached?

Providing constructive criticism, negative feedback or challenging someone's action is difficult at any time. There may be appropriate communication and management channels through which this is best conducted such as through appraisal or management supervision. However, as the scenario above has highlighted, there are times when it may be appropriate to provide that feedback yourself. This is important for effective leadership. As highlighted above, providing this feedback can involve the following:

- Questioning what happened and hearing the other person's side of the story.
- Considering and exploring alternative possibilities.
- Attempting to consider the person's perspective and if they had a rationale for what they did.
- Tactfully sharing experiences and alternatives.

A leader's role in creating and managing change is particularly important within nursing (DH 2006a). This is especially relevant within the NHS. Structures and process are often in flux as the health services respond to the changing health needs of the population, developing technology, innovation and resource pressures. Brimblecombe (2009) highlights that it is important for mental health nurses to consider change in line with the values of mental health nursing and the needs and wishes of service users and their families. As a mental health nurse, you may be involved in driving and creating changes within the practice environment. However, change can be unsettling for many so you also have a key role in supporting other members of staff through this process. Changes can be particularly difficult for some people who use services. Therefore, helping the individual deal with this change will be part of leading healthcare delivery.

Williams (2004) reviewed the literature relating to leadership development in organisations and found there were some strategies that were used by effective leaders to enable change to happen. These included the following:

- Identifying others whose opinion is valued/followed in a team.
- Involving people through small groups in implementing a change.
- Developing ways for those involved to share and reflect on their experiences.
- Identifying and employing particular tools and techniques such as following an

assessment, planning, implementation and evaluation cycle.

- Identifying goals that are small and achievable.
- Focusing on action.

As the first part of this chapter highlighted, there are core areas of nursing practice where leadership is inherent including decision making, innovation and coordinating care. The community is increasingly offering opportunities for newly qualified mental health nurses. Working in this environment often involves working autonomously and effectively managing your own work load. One of the most common methods of organising workloads and delivering care in the community is through case management. The following section explores case management in community care and links this with leadership skills.

Case management

What is case management?

Case management is a means of adapting help to meet individuals' specific needs by allocating responsibility for assessment and coordination of services with one individual worker or team (Oynett 1998). The core responsibilities of a case manager may be seen to generally reflect the nursing process in terms of assessment, planning, implementation, monitoring and review. There are a number of different models of case management which might structure the particular approach taken within a given team. The aims of case management are to ensure that service users are provided with the services that they need in a coordinated and effective way. Case management is one of the most common ways of leading care in mental health practice.

Case management has emerged from the growth in community-based mental health services. More recently, CPA policy identified the need to integrate the CPA with case management (DH 1999). Community nurses (alongside other professionals) will therefore be acting as care coordinators or case managers for a number of people using services at any one time.

Case management is increasingly being recognised in the wider policy relating to health care and nursing as the most valuable way of organising care delivery in the community. This literature suggests that case management involves clear decision making, articulating a rationale for decisions made and negotiating with other care providers and deliverers (including other organisations). The case management role may also include teaching others, which could be service users, families, students, junior staff or practitioners from other organisations (DH 2004). A socially inclusive approach to care management was emphasised to enable individuals to access or maintain valued roles and activities within the community (DH 2004, 2006c, 2008). Some policies acknowledge that such a role in case management might involve practice development and service improvement (DH 2006b). This is also underpinned by a greater emphasis on the opportunities for nursing leadership, through coordinating (and commissioning) care (DH 2006a).

Case management and mental health

Following the development of community-based services for the delivery of mental health care, a number of models of case management have been developed in mental health:

- Standard case management (brokerage and clinical case management).
- Rehabilitation orientated (strengths and rehabilitation models).
- Intensive case management (intensive and assertive models).

The different models of case management have provided some structure to therapeutic activity in specific teams. This reflects the different expectations, philosophies and skills that a professional may use within each approach. For instance, Mueser et al (1998) suggested that clinical case management has had a greater focus on providing education and psychological-based support for service users. The strengths model of case management involves working within the strengths approach, as advocated by Charles Rapp, and accessing community resources. With the possible exception of assertive outreach services within contemporary mental health care, the majority of practitioners might claim to use a number of different models or

---

 Activity

You are most likely to encounter a case management approach when on placement with a community team such as an older persons' community team, early intervention in pyschosis team, community mental health team or rehabilitation and recovery team (see Ch. 4 for details on these services). While in one or more of these areas, talk to the team members about what they perceive are the benefits and challenges of a case management approach. Additionally, ask them about the skills that they use in order to manage the time and resources that they have for their case loads. After the discussion, consider:

1. What have you learnt from this discussion?
2. What are the implications of this for your future practice?

You might also want to think about what, if any, model of case management outlined below you have observed in the team.

approaches to inform their practice rather than operate within a specific model of case management.

Evaluation

Case management has helped practitioners establish relationships with individuals living in the community and has therefore been shown to impact on the contact people have with services (Marshall et al 2011). Simpson et al (2003) provide a review of the literature evaluating models of case management. They highlighted some difficulties in drawing definitive conclusions about the benefits of case management due to a lack of robust research studies in the area. However, the paper suggested that the content of sessions between service users and case managers contributes to improvements in outcomes rather than the number of sessions. This is important as one of the challenges that case management has brought is the potentially large case loads that community nurses work with. This requires a practitioner to use effective organisational and time management skills as well as being able to assess, negotiate and prioritise the support both they and others provide to the people they are working with. Ryan et al (1994) found that interventions promoted by the strengths model of case management had a greater effect on promoting social inclusion and improving individuals' skills to live independently than any others.

Working with other organisations

Case management often involves working with organisations that deliver care or social support outside of the NHS. (Chapter 1 introduced multidisciplinary and partnership working in mental health care.) These organisations may be charitable, social or private and could include establishments such as housing associations, hostel providers or hospitals run by private companies. The ability to develop effective partnerships with service users, families and non-statutory organisations has been identified as an essential skill for mental health nurses (DH 2001, 2004, 2006a). There is some differentiation between partnership and interagency working. Interagency working refers to interactions between different organisations for the delivery of care. This may relate to a specific aspect of care delivery or a defined period where professionals coming from different organisations may work together towards a common goal.

Partnership working

What is partnership working?

A partnership is defined as a relationship between parties or more than one agency. The concept of partnership implies an equal relationship. In order for this to be achieved, decisions are made jointly and power is shared. Partnership working is integrated within the delivery of mental health services through the NHS and Community Care Act (1990) which created provisions for health and social care services to work together and to ensure joint working was organised at a more strategic level. Partnerships may include strategic and financial agreement at the level of the commissioning of services. It can also be incorporated into organisational structure. For instance, some trusts are jointly health and social care trusts. In order to ensure effective and efficient partnership working, structures may be joined such as one IT or joint paperwork frameworks (which includes the CPA). However, this doesn't occur in all organisations which can sometimes be a barrier to communication.

Equality can be difficult to achieve within partnerships. This is particularly evident when considering the development of partnership with service users and families where mental health professionals possess more power within the decision-making process. It can also be hard to escape the perceptions of professional hierarchies and the institutional power base that accompanies this when working with establishments outside the NHS.

Different organisations often have different unwritten codes about the way they work and this informs the organisational culture. Each agency may also have specific aims and goals which will ultimately work towards offering good quality care and support to people who use their service but these may differ in their philosophy, structure and language. Understanding and identifying these differences can be really important for a nurse working with other organisations to promote working together efficiently.

The section above highlighted the importance of this in terms of the delivery of mental health care. Through this and the reflective exercise, some of the challenges of working in partnership have been recognised.

Effective partnership working is supported by the following:

- Understanding the role and function of teams (both your own and the team that you are working with).
- Understanding professional roles and boundaries.
- Working positively with any difference in aspiration or conflicts of interest.
- A supporting infrastructure.
- Open communication.
- Integrating training and support.
- Clear strategic objectives.

Learning to work effectively with other agencies is essential within contemporary mental health services.

(•) Reflection point

Reflecting on your practice experiences so far, identify a situation where you have been involved in decision making in mental health practice (this may be as an observer or as part of the contributions made to an individual's care). Through the development of a reflective piece, examine:

1. Who was involved in the decision?
2. What organisations were involved?
3. Was there any difference in perceptions?
4. Did you notice anything about who seemed to have the most say?
5. What implications does this have for partnership working?

(◉) Activity

While on your next placement, identify agencies or organisations that your practice area works with. Make a list.

Pick two organisations and try to arrange an insight visit or opportunity to meet with one of their workers to talk through what their service provides. After this visit, think about:

1. What, if any, are the differences in how the organisation is structured?
2. What is the aim or philosophy of the service? Are there any similarities or differences with that of the NHS?
3. What challenges do the other organisations identify for working with the NHS?
4. How can effective communication between the agencies be promoted?

Most decisions in mental health practice, particularly in community settings, involve different professions, service users and people working for different organisations.

The activities above may help you to achieve your NMC pre-registration competencies.

Nursing careers

The Chief Nursing Officer's review of mental health nursing expresses a commitment to nursing careers which offer a wide range of options, including leadership, for the provision of excellent care (DH 2006b). This chapter has considered that leadership is part of delivering person-centred effective nursing care (Kitson 2001, DH 2008). However, there are opportunities within nursing to more formally develop the leadership aspect of the role. Figure 14.1 demonstrates some of the career structures that enable this. Nursing is evolving rapidly with new roles and opportunities arising. It is worth exploring the advanced and leadership roles that are linked to your service areas while on placement to keep abreast of developments and explore potential career pathways.

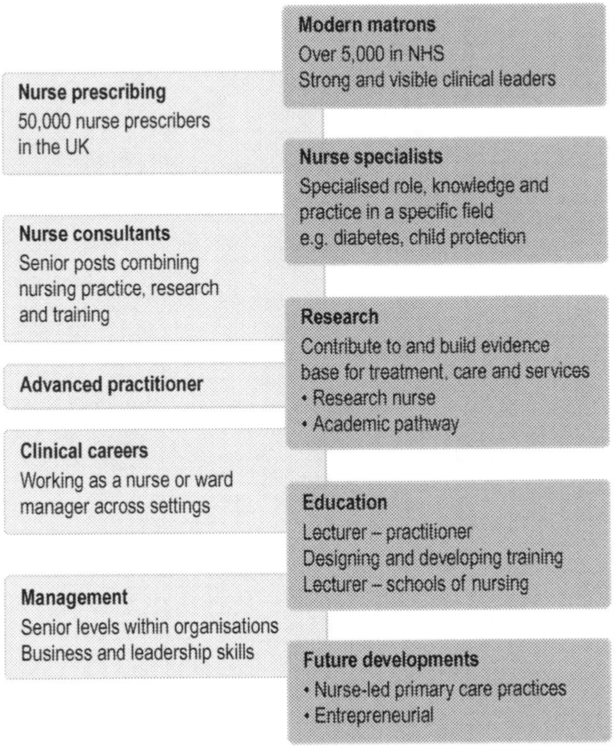

Modern matrons
Over 5,000 in NHS
Strong and visible clinical leaders

Nurse prescribing
50,000 nurse prescribers in the UK

Nurse specialists
Specialised role, knowledge and practice in a specific field
e.g. diabetes, child protection

Nurse consultants
Senior posts combining nursing practice, research and training

Research
Contribute to and build evidence base for treatment, care and services
• Research nurse
• Academic pathway

Advanced practitioner

Clinical careers
Working as a nurse or ward manager across settings

Education
Lecturer – practitioner
Designing and developing training
Lecturer – schools of nursing

Management
Senior levels within organisations
Business and leadership skills

Future developments
• Nurse-led primary care practices
• Entrepreneurial

Fig 14.1 Career opportunities in nursing

References

Antrobus, S., Kitson, A., 1999. Nursing leadership; influencing and shaping health policy and nursing practice. Journal of Advanced Nursing 29 (3), 746–753.

Brimblecombe, N., 2009a. Leadership and management. In: Callaghan, P., Playle, J., Cooper, L, (Eds), Mental health nursing skills. Oxford University Press, Oxford.

Department of Health, 1999. Effective care co-ordination in mental health services: modernising the Care Programme Approach. HMSO, London.

Department of Health, 2001. Journey to recovery: the government's vision for mental health care. HMSO, London.

Department of Health, 2004. Ten essential shared capabilities: a framework for the whole mental health workforce. HMSO, London.

Department of Health, 2006a. Modernising nursing careers, setting the direction. HMSO, London.

Department of Health, 2006b. From values to action: Chief Nursing Officer's review of mental health nursing. HMSO, London.

Department of Health, 2006c. Our health, our care, our say: a new direction for community services. A brief guide, HMSO, London.

Department of Health, 2008. High quality care for all: the next stage review. HMSO, London.

Kitson, A., 2001. Nursing leadership: bringing caring back to the future. Quality in Health Care 10, 79–84.

Kotter, J., 1990a. A course for change: how leadership differs from management. Free Press, New York.

Kotter, J., 1990b. What leaders really do. Harvard Business Review 68 (3), 103–111.

Marshall, M., Gray, A., Lockwood, A., Green, R., 2011. Case management for people with severe mental disorders. Cochrane Database of Systematic Reviews(4) Art. No.: CD000050. doi:10.1002/14651858.CD000050. pub2.

Mueser, K., Bond, G., Drake, R., Resnick, S., 1998. Models of community care for severe mental illness: a review of research on case management. Schizophrenia Bulletin 24 (1), 37–74.

Nursing and Midwifery Council, 2008. Code of professional conduct. NMC, London.

Oynett, S., 1998. Case management in mental health. Chapman Hall, London.

Ramsden, P., 1998. Learning to lead in higher education. Routledge, London.

Ryan, C., Sherman, P., Judd, C., 1994. Accounting for case manager effects in the evaluation of mental health services. Journal of Consulting and Clinical Psychology 62, 965–974.

Simpson, A., Miller, C., Bowers, L., 2003. Case management models and the Care Programme Approach: how to make the CPA effective and credible. Journal of Psychiatric and Mental Health Nursing 10 (4), 472–483.

Williams, S., 2004. Evidence of the contribution leadership development for professional groups makes in driving their organisations forward for NHS leadership. Centre Henley Management College, Henley.

Williamson, G., Jenkinson, T., Proctor-Childs, T., 2008. Contexts of contemporary nursing, 2nd ed. Learning Matters, Exeter.

Further reading

Brimblecome, N., 2009. Leadership and management. In: Callaghan, P., Playle, J., Cooper, L. (Eds.), Mental health nursing skills. Oxford University Press, Oxford.

Department of Health, 2006a. Modernising nursing careers, setting the direction. HMSO, London.

Department of Health, 2006b. From values to action: Chief Nursing Officer's review of mental health nursing. HMSO, London.

Websites

Mental health nursing careers, http://www.nhscareers.nhs.uk/details/Default.aspx?Id=122 (accessed June 2011).

A guide to roles in mental health, http://www.mind.org.uk/help/research_and_policy/whos_who_in_mental_health_a_brief_guide (accessed June 2011).

Section 3. Reflecting on practice learning

Introduction

The following chapters will help you to apply key areas of learning to extended clinical case studies and challenging situations. You will be encouraged to test your knowledge throughout this section and consider the scenarios from the perspectives of all the people involved. It will also give examples of challenges students commonly experience in mental health placements. You will be prompted to use the knowledge you have gained from this book, the recommended reading and your placement experiences to consider how you might respond to each of these case studies and situations. You may want to discuss the scenarios with your peers, mentor or personal tutor to gain their perspectives and advice. There is not necessarily a right or wrong answer to the issues raised in this section. However, you should draw upon the theory, skills and extended reading identified in this book along with your experiences in practice to inform your responses.

15   The service user experience

CHAPTER AIMS

- To gain an understanding of the service user experience of mental health services
- To engage in reflection on learning in practice and from practice in relation to the service user experience

Introduction

The following case studies describe three different experiences of accessing mental health services. The questions that follow each section aim to prompt you to apply your reading, experience and discussion to a clinical situation. You may already have this knowledge or you may need to do some additional research. The activity boxes in case studies 1 and 2 will direct you to sources of information which will help you to learn or reflect upon how you might respond to a situation or manage the clinical scenario. However, in case study 3 you are encouraged to use your own research skills to seek out the information required.

Case study 1: young male experiencing his first psychotic episode

This case study will focus on a young male who experiences a psychotic episode for the first time. When reading this case study, you should consider the following key areas of learning and think about how you would apply them to your own clinical practice, including how they help you to achieve your practice competencies to become a registered nurse:

- Communication skills.
- Engagement.
- The therapeutic relationship.
- Assessment.
- Risk assessment.
- Care planning.
- Working with families.
- Responding to people who experience unusual beliefs.
- Mental health law.
- Personal safety.

9.15 a.m. Monday

A phone call from the GP to the crisis intervention and home treatment team:

GP: Hi, I need an urgent assessment of one of my patients, Christopher Ellis. His mother has been in and out of the surgery for the last 4 days saying that he is acting oddly and won't leave his room. He hasn't eaten for the past week and, as far as his mum knows, he hasn't even been to the toilet. It all came to a head last night when his dad banged his door down and they ended up in a physical fight. Can you get out to him today?

CPN: Yes, that will be fine but we will need some more detailed information from you first.

 Activity

1. What additional information would you and your mentor need from the GP in order to inform your approach to the initial visit?

2. How would you and your mentor approach your initial visit taking into consideration how Christopher and his family may be feeling?

3. What would be the priorities for the first visit?

4. What might you discuss or clarify with your mentor before the visit in relation to your role and learning?

You may want to refer to the sections on assessment (Ch. 8) and forming therapeutic relationships (Ch. 7) to help you with these questions. The students' top tips in Chapter 4 may also help you to think about what role you could have in this scenario and how you might approach this with your mentor to achieve your learning goals.

11.30 a.m. Monday
You arrive at Christopher's home with your mentor. Christopher's mum opens the door. She has obviously been crying and does not look like she has slept. Your mentor introduces you both and you enter the house.

 Activity

5. What factors should you consider in terms of your personal safety when visiting someone in their own home for the first time?

6. How might you greet Christopher's mum once you have been introduced?

The section on practicalities in Chapter 5 will help you with this one. There should also be a policy relating to this in your practice area which you should read before going out on home visits, even if you are with your mentor. You could also look at the communication section in Chapter 6 to help you consider how you might enhance your approachability when meeting Christopher's mum.

Your mentor explains to Christopher's mum that her GP has referred Christopher to the service and that you are both here to find out more about what has been going on in order to agree on the best way forward. His mum immediately appears relieved, bursts into tears and thanks your mentor for agreeing to help. You offer her a tissue from your bag which she takes and she smiles at you. Your mentor begins the assessment process.

 Activity

7. What questions might your mentor ask to initiate the assessment process?

8. What style of questioning might be appropriate at this stage?

Chapter 8 on assessment will give you some ideas about how to work through this scenario. You may also have observed your mentor or other professionals in practice and learnt from their approach.

You learn from Christopher's mum that he has been smoking cannabis on and off for the past 4 years. She tells you that although she doesn't agree with it, it doesn't seem to do him any harm and she appreciates that most of his friends are also doing it. Over the past month he seemed to be smoking more and she had a hard time getting him out of bed in the morning to go to his job in the local call centre. He had been late so many times that he got the sack and hasn't made any effort to look for something else.

His Dad has been getting more and more frustrated with him and they have been arguing all the time. This led to Christopher retreating to his room and the smell of cannabis was constantly coming from his door. Last week Christopher's mum convinced him to let her in to his room to change the sheets. She was shocked because all his electrical gadgets had been taken to pieces and were scattered all over the floor. Christopher told her that they were all malfunctioning because of aliens attempting to communicate with him through his TV, iPod and computer. She initially thought he was joking, but when she returned from home the next day he had also taken the microwave in the kitchen to pieces and made a start on the downstairs TV. His Dad was furious and that was when they went to see Dr Ascot at the GP surgery. She described things as going from bad to worse since then:

> Christopher has locked himself in his room and hasn't had a scrap to eat. He keeps telling me that the food is contaminated! God knows where he is going to the toilet because he hasn't been out of there in days. Last night his Dad got to the end of his tether and banged the door down. Christopher went crazy, shouting about the aliens and that they were coming for him. He pushed his Dad out of the door and hasn't been out again since. I'm so worried about what he might do to himself in there.

Activity

9. How might you initially respond to Christopher's mum?
10. What are your impressions of what is going on for Christopher?
11. Thinking about the Stress Vulnerability Model, what might be the factors which are increasing Christopher's stress and vulnerability at this time?
12. What would be your next course of action?

It seems like Christopher's mum is highly distressed by the situation and would benefit initially from reassurance and support. Additional reading, such as Gamble and Brennan (2000) and Chapter 10 on working with people who experience voices and unusual beliefs, might help you understand what might be going on for Christopher and inform your decision around your course of action.

You and your mentor discuss your next steps and decide to try and talk to Christopher. You agree that two people may be intimidating so your mentor initially approaches him and you stay with his mum to provide comfort and reassurance. Your mentor returns after 15 minutes and tells you that Christopher hasn't responded to her at all although she can hear him pacing in his bedroom.

Activity

13. What other approaches might you suggest to encourage Christopher to engage with your mentor?
14. What are the risks that are currently present?

The document *Keys to Engagement* (1998) published by the Sainsbury Centre for Mental Health and Chapter 7 on forming therapeutic relationships might offer you some ideas on approaches to working with Christopher. You could discuss with your peers what risks are present in this scenario. Chapter 12 will also help you to identify the risks and possible ways of working with them in a way that is therapeutic.

You suggest to your mentor that you could try writing a note to Christopher telling him who you are and that you would like to speak with him about his worries and fears. You could say that you might be able to help and that you will come back this afternoon to see if he would like to speak with you. Your mentor agrees that this is a good option as Christopher may be suspicious of her motives and finding it difficult to trust her. His mum agrees with the plan and takes your contact details in case anything happens in the meantime.

3.30 p.m. Monday

You and your mentor return to the house. Christopher's mum tells you that she has heard him continually talking in his room. Your mentor approaches his room again and he opens the door slightly. He is sitting on the floor and your mentor also sits down on the other side of the door. She introduces herself and they talk for some time. Christopher tells her in detail about his fears for his safety as the aliens will be coming for him at 6.30 that evening. He tells her that he would rather die than let them take him because they have told him what they will do to his brain. He is highly distressed, scared and speaking very quickly. Your mentor talks with him about going into hospital as a

place of safety to get help with the thoughts and beliefs that he has. Christopher becomes angry with this and accuses your mentor of being part of the plot to get him out of his room. He slams and locks the door.

Activity

15. What are your concerns about Christopher's level of risk in light of gathering his perspective?
16. What action do you think your mentor will need to take as a result of his response?

It may be helpful to talk with a few mental health practitioners and find out how they would respond to this scenario. We often find that different practitioners view levels of risk differently and therefore would respond differently. It can be helpful to consider what influences the practitioners' responses and discuss the subjective nature of assessing risk.

You and your mentor agree that you will need to initiate a Mental Health Act assessment in order to ensure that Christopher and his family are not placed at further risk. You discuss this with Christopher's mum and inform her of the process that will be followed.

Activity

17. What would be the purpose and rationale for a Mental Health Act assessment in this scenario?
18. What would be your mentor's role and responsibilities in organising and carrying out the Mental Health Act assessment?

19. How might the Mental Health Act assessment be carried out in a way that is least distressing for Christopher?

20. What could be the possible outcomes of the Mental Health Act assessment?

Look at the practitioners' guides to mental health law referenced in Chapter 3. Once you have read some of this material, examine with your peers how you think this might apply to Christopher's situation using the questions above to prompt your discussions.

8.30 p.m. Monday

Christopher is admitted to hospital on Section 2 of the Mental Health Act for assessment. On arrival at the ward he is taken to a side room and given a drink. A nurse sits with him until he is settled. He is given some medication to help him sleep and will be seen by the doctor in the morning. Christopher remains scared and requires a great deal of reassurance from staff about his safety.

Activity

21. What type of medication may be helpful for Christopher in light of his distress and difficulty sleeping?

Chapter 9 looks at supporting people to make choices about their treatment and will help you to identify the type of medication that Christopher might benefit from. You may also want to look this medication up in the *British National Formulary* (Royal Pharmaceutical Society 2010) to give you more information on the dose and possible side effects.

Case study 2: a 57-year-old female who has had long-term contact with mental health services

This case study will focus on the experiences of a 57-year-old female who has been in contact with mental health services for many years. When reading this case study, you should consider the following key areas of learning and think about how you would apply them to your clinical practice:

- Recovery and social inclusion.
- Values-based practice and self-awareness.
- Engagement.
- Communication skills.
- The therapeutic relationship.
- Risk management.
- Challenging negative attitudes in teams.
- Coping skills.
- Physical health problems.
- Working with people who are diagnosed with personality disorder.

Setting the scene

You are on placement at a residential rehabilitation unit in the voluntary sector. The unit offers support to people who have been in contact with mental health services for many years and aims to facilitate the move to independent living. You arrive at the unit for the first day and you are greeted by your mentor who introduces you to a number of the service users who are residents on the unit. She encourages you to spend the first week getting to know the residents and the routines of the unit. She advises you to avoid reading the residents' medical notes before you have had a chance to meet them and to spend as much time as possible engaging with them.

Activity

1. What might be the rationale for a service which aims to support people with long-term mental health problems to move into their own accommodation?
2. Why might your mentor encourage you not to read the residents' medical notes before you have met them?

Chapter 1 describes the history of mental health services and the changes that have occurred over time to ensure that mental health care is delivered in the least restrictive environment. Reading this chapter will help to inform your answer to question 1.

Chapters 6 and 7 both identify the importance of being aware of prejudices and the importance of displaying a non-judgemental attitude towards others. These chapters will help you to think about how reading a service user's notes before meeting them might influence your opinion of them and your ability to demonstrate these key qualities which facilitate the building of a therapeutic relationship.

Week 1

You initially spend a great deal of time with 57-year-old Mary who is preparing to move out over the next month. You begin general chit chat and start to get to know her. She tells you that she is looking forward to having her own place as it is 16 years since she has lived alone. You immediately like Mary and find it easy to talk to her. You plan to go shopping together for the things that she needs for her new home and help her to complete forms for reassessment of her benefits. You notice that Mary is often breathless when walking short distances and is significantly overweight. You attempt to initiate a conversation with Mary about this

but she changes the subject to a TV programme she has watched.

Activity

3. What approaches are being used here to facilitate engagement with Mary?
4. Why might Mary be reluctant to discuss her physical health with you and what is your role in promoting physical health?
5. What might be the therapeutic benefits of the relationship that you are building with Mary?

Chapter 7 and further reading such as Callaghan et al (2009) will help you to think about what is going on within the interaction between you and Mary. You will also find the information in Chapter 6 on health promotion helpful to understand Mary's reluctance to discuss her physical health.

You attend handover for the first time and feed back to the team on your activities with Mary. You are surprised when a couple of the team members begin to laugh. You ask them what they are laughing at.

– Ah, don't worry about it love, we were just laughing because she always takes advantage of the students. She's a manipulative one that one, and you need to watch her. She'll have you doing everything for her before you know it. You do know about her history, don't you?

– No, my mentor advised me to get to know the residents before I read their notes.

– Well, about 30 years ago she set fire to her house with herself and her kids in it. Ended up at one of those high-secure hospitals. Never been allowed to see her kids since. She'll be on one of those Home Office sections for the rest of her life I reckon.

Activity

6. What is your response to this information?

7. How might it influence how you work with Mary from now on?

8. How do you feel about the team member's attitude towards Mary?

The section on values-based practice in Chapter 3 might help you to reflect on how you feel towards the team's response. You may also want to discuss this with your student colleagues and identify how you might respond to them if you were placed in this situation in practice.

You decide to write a reflective piece for your portfolio to consider how this information has impacted on you. You discuss this with your mentor who encourages you to think critically about the way other team members respond to Mary in order to understand their perspective and identify how you may challenge it in the future. Your mentor supports you to continue in your work with Mary and you discuss what you have learnt about the values and skills which underpin the building of therapeutic relationships. She also reminds you that you will only have a limited time to work with Mary and asks you to think about how you will manage that towards the end of your placement.

Activity

9. Why might other team members be responding to Mary in this way?

10. How might you challenge these attitudes:
   a. as a student
   b. as a qualified nurse?

11. What are the values and skills that underpin the building of therapeutic relationships that your mentor is referring to?

12. How might you prepare for ending the therapeutic relationship?

Draw upon your previous reading on forming therapeutic relationships and discussion with your mentor to consider the ways you might prepare for ending therapeutic relationships.

Week 6

Mary has moved into her new home and you are continuing to visit her as part of her care plan to facilitate her transition. You notice that she appears anxious and is continually asking you for reassurance about day-to-day things that she would normally take in her stride. When you leave, she continually calls the unit and asks to speak with you for long periods of time. If you make attempts to end the phone call, she tells you that she isn't coping and can only feel calm when she is speaking to you.

Activity

13. Why might Mary be finding the transition to independent living anxiety provoking?

14. What concerns might you have about how Mary is responding to you and the requests she is making on your time?

15. How might you manage this situation?

This one is difficult and would need to take into account Mary's specific needs and the approach the team adopts to supporting people to move on. Discuss with your mentor how this situation would be managed in your current placement area. Chat with your student colleages to find out if their placements would respond differently.

Week 7

You visit Mary at home as planned and feel increasingly concerned about how she is coping. Her home is messy and she has out-of-date food in her cupboards and fridge. You remind Mary that you will be leaving the placement in 3 weeks and she becomes very distressed. She tells you that you are the only person who she can trust and that she doesn't feel she can cope without your support. You try to reassure Mary but this doesn't seem to work. You return to the unit and immediately seek support from one of the nurses.

> – *I'm really concerned about Mary. She seems to be becoming more and more dependent on me no matter how hard I try to reassure her that she is doing really well on her own.*
> – *It takes a lot for Mary to trust someone and she will be upset that you are leaving. This is her way of telling you how much you mean to her. People with personality disorder often behave in this way because of past relationships.*
> – *It feels like she is forcing me to push her away because I just can't meet her demands.*
> – *Perhaps you could spend your last few weeks looking at her coping skills so that she knows she has other options other than support from you? We could do some more joint visits as well to remind her that there is support available from the whole team.*
> – *Yeah that could work well. I will give it a go.*

🔊 Activity

16. Why might Mary be expressing her distress in this way?

17. How might you approach working with Mary to enhance her coping skills?

18. How might other members of the multidisciplinary team help support Mary to cope in her new home?

Chapter 11 will assist you to consider how you might support Mary to cope with her anxiety and develop a sense of personal control to help reduce her dependence on you.

End of placement

You reflect with your mentor on how you have worked with Mary and what you have learnt to inform your future practice. You spend your final visit with Mary at the local café which serves her favourite cheesecake. You thank Mary for the time you have spent with her and wish her the best for the future. You feel confident that she will be well supported by the team and that her care plan has been reviewed in light of her new goals for the future.

Case study 3: experience of a young female student nurse who has been referred to mental health services

This case study will focus on the experiences of a young female student nurse who has been referred to a mental health nurse working in a primary care setting by her GP. When reading this case study, you should consider the following key areas of learning and think about how you would apply them to your clinical practice:

- Medication management.
- Assessment.
- Risk assessment and management.

- Coping skills.
- Reduced levels of activity.
- Recovery and social inclusion.
- Stigma and discrimination.
- Values-based practice and self-awareness.
- Personal wellbeing.

Setting the scene

Anna has been seeing her GP, for the past 6 months, who has diagnosed her with mild anxiety and depression. He has prescribed sertraline which she takes when her mood is low but not on a daily basis as prescribed. Anna is a student nurse and has been finding it increasingly difficult to go to her placement and attend lectures. She has spoken to her personal tutor, about the difficulties she is having, who is supporting her to continue but has raised concerns about her ability to manage the stress and demands of the course. Anna is very concerned that she will be thrown off the course and that peers, mentors and tutors will perceive her as incapable or unsafe. She is therefore reluctant to tell her mentors and peers about her mental health problem which is leading to people perceiving her as unsociable and not interested in her studies.

Activity

1. How might anxiety and depression be impacting on Anna's ability to engage in her nurse education?
2. What is sertraline and how might Anna's way of taking it be influencing its efficacy?
3. What do you think about how Anna is managing the situation in terms of disclosing her problems to peers and mentors?
4. How would you feel if you were in a similar situation and how might you manage it?

Anna's mood continues to deteriorate. She stops attending lectures and communicating with her personal tutor. She spends her days at home and is beginning to feel scared to leave the house. She feels guilty and believes she is a failure but is unable to take any action to help herself. She begins to have thoughts of ending her life due to the hopelessness she feels with her situation. She finds her sadness is relieved when she digs her nails into her arms. This helps her expel her anger with herself. Her boyfriend, who is beginning to feel frustrated and impatient, forces her to go back to her GP. She tells her GP about the thoughts she is having. In response, he refers her to a mental health nurse who is working in primary care for assessment.

Activity

5. What are your views regarding risk in relation to Anna's current mood, thoughts and behaviour?
6. From a cognitive behavioural therapy perspective, how would you describe the way Anna currently copes with her problems?
7. How might the mental health nurse approach the assessment process?
8. What might be the mental health nurse's possible course of action following the assessment?

Anna attends the assessment and discusses in depth how her thoughts and feelings are impacting on her behaviour. She is able to identify her negative thinking patterns and recognise how she is managing her mood and anxiety in an unhelpful way which is leading to further deterioration in her mental health. They talk about her suicidal thoughts and Anna is able to see that this is a response to her feeling that she has no other way out. She is reassured by the mental health nurse's plan to see her weekly for the next 6 weeks to focus on how she can make changes and alter her current way of thinking.

 Activity

> 9. What are the negative thinking patterns that Anna might be experiencing?
> 10. How might her thoughts of suicide be interpreted by the mental health nurse?
> 11. What type of interventions might be helpful when working with Anna to address her reduced activity levels?

Anna receives an e-mail from herpersonal tutor asking her to get in touch and expressing concerns about her poor attendance and lack of communication. Anna deletes the e-mail and decides that the

 Activity

> 12. How is the way Anna responds to this e-mail linked to her negative thinking style and unhelpful behavioural response?
> 13. How accurate do you think Anna's perception is of attitudes to mental health problems within nursing as a profession?
> 14. How might the mental health nurse and Anna's personal tutor work with Anna to support her to continue with her course?
> 15. What role might education and employment play in Anna's recovery from her mental health problem?

tutor will think she is not able to continue and therefore there is no point in discussing her recent appointment and plans with him. She also thinks that others will agree that nurses should not have mental health problems and, therefore, the Nursing and Midwifery Council (NMC) would not allow her to register.

Anna discusses the e-mail from her personal tutor with the mental health nurse. They identify that responding to this should be a priority for the first stage of change, with her overall goal being to return to university and complete her nurse education. Anna goes home and writes the e-mail, explaining her circumstances and the help she is receiving. She arranges to meet with her tutor to discuss her options and gain accurate information which may challenge the assumptions she is making about how the NMC will respond to her problems. Anna and her tutor agree that she would benefit from a short break from the course due to the amount she has missed but with a view to returning in a few months. Anna agrees to communicate frequently with her personal tutor and share with him the work she has been doing on relapse prevention so that he can support her during times of stress. Anna is aware that this has been documented in her file and, at times, she does feel concerned about people seeing it and judging her.

 Activity

> 16. How might meeting with her tutor influence Anna's negative thinking patterns and unhelpful behaviours?
> 17. How is the tutor's response conducive to Anna's social inclusion and recovery?
> 18. Why might Anna still hold concerns about others judging her as a result of her mental health problems?

References

Callaghan, P., Playle, J., Cooper, L., 2009. Mental health nursing skills. Oxford University Press, Oxford.

Gamble, C., Brennan, G., 2000. Working with serious mental illness: a manual for clinical practice. Baillière Tindall, Edinburgh.

Royal Pharmaceutical Society, 2010. British national formulary 61. Pharmaceutical Press, London.

Sainsbury Centre for Mental Health, 1998. Keys to engagement. SCMH, London.

Websites

British National Formulary 61: http://bnf.org/bnf/current/ (accessed June 2011).

16 Turning challenges into opportunities in mental health placements

CHAPTER AIMS

- To explore challenges student nurses experience in mental health placements
- To consider possible options that student nurses can take in experiencing these challenges

Introduction

This chapter will give examples of challenges students commonly experience in mental health placements. You will be prompted to use the knowledge you have gained from this book, the recommended reading and your placement experiences to reflect upon how you might respond to each of these situations. You may want to discuss the scenarios with your peers, mentor or personal tutor to gain their perspectives and advice. The scenarios are based on actual experiences of student nurses in practice.

Clinical challenges

1. I have been given a man to work with on my own by my mentor. She would like me to help him with his low motivation and reduced activity. The problem is, everything I suggest he just dismisses or says he isn't interested. I'm getting nowhere and I'm feeling like I might as well give up.

2. My mentor has told me to spend time on the ward in the communal areas getting to know the service users but no one seems to want to talk to me. They are all in their own world as far as I can see and I don't know how to get in there.

3. I've been visiting a woman for the last 3 weeks and things seemed to be going well. Last week I got held up at another visit and was 5 minutes late. She was fuming when I arrived. She refused to let me in, and by the time I got back to the office she had contacted my mentor to complain about me. I was so embarrassed.

Professional issues

1. I was spending time with one of the service users I have been keyworking with my mentor yesterday and she was really opening up. We were talking about her future and that was when she told me she didn't see a future for herself. She said she knows that she will

kill herself one day but told me not to tell anyone because they will overreact.

2. I was in the car with my mentor who I've been getting along with really well. She started to tell me about all these problems she is having at home and started to cry. She said she isn't coping at all and finding it really hard to do her job.

3. I was on the ward yesterday and I saw this health care assistant (HCA) really taunting one of the service users. I could see she was getting more and more angry but I didn't know what to say. Eventually the service user blew up and started shouting at the HCA. The alarms went off and loads of staff appeared to restrain her. She got even angrier and hit out. Eventually, they had to give her some medication to calm her down. The HCA didn't say anything about the lead up to it and said it was just out of the blue.

Learning opportunities

1. I'm on placement in the assertive outreach, and about three-quarters of the service users don't want me to visit them with my mentor. My mentor says we have to respect their choice, which I understand, but I'm spending more than half my time sitting in the car. I'm worried I won't meet my competencies.

2. My mentor is the team leader on the ward and is too busy to spend time with me. She's really nice and keeps telling me I'm doing fine but I feel that I need more guidance and support. Also, how is she going to sign my competencies if she hasn't seen me practise?

3. I'm really not sure what I'm going to get from this placement as all I see the nurses do is sit in the office doing paperwork. That's not what I came into

nursing for and I'm disappointed that it seems to take up so much of their time.

Possible answers

Consider the following possible answers to these experiences and discuss with your personal tutor or mentor in practice.

Clinical challenges

1. The key to this scenario is finding the service user's internal motivation. This refers to the things that interest, excite or stimulate him. This may be something simple like a music artist or particular film. Once this has been identified, you can build upon this to offer suggestions in line with his interests. Often people mistake low motivation for a genuine lack of interest in the suggestions you are offering. The best place to start is with the person's history – what did they enjoy before they struggled with their mental health problem? This type of work can be frustrating as you may feel you are not getting very far. It is important to seek support which will allow you to express your frustrations in order to stick with the person and continue to show your interest in them. It is also essential to recognise small signs of improvement and identify the impact the little things can have on a person's overall quality of life.

2. People who are admitted to an acute ward are often preoccupied by their distress and may find it hard to initiate conversation. They may also be suspicious of who you are and your rationale for being there. A good place to start is with a neutral topic or activity that allows the person to get to know you and begin to trust you. This might involve commenting on a TV programme or inviting someone to play a game. This can often have a domino

effect as others begin to see that you are an approachable person who is interested in spending time with them without a negative ulterior motive.

3. A common theme with people who experience mental health problems is the existence of negative relationships with people who they should have been able to trust. Being a little late for an appointment may seem insignificant to you but may imply your lack of commitment or unreliability to the service user. It is important to be consistent and to ensure that you live up to promises or arrangements you make in order to encourage the person to trust you.

Professional issues

1. In these circumstances, you would have a responsibility to pass this information on to your mentor as the service user is expressing feelings which may lead to significant harm or suicide. In order to prevent this situation, it is important to discuss with the service user the limitations of confidentiality from the outset so that they are clear you are not able to withhold such information. You can then remind them of this if such a situation arises. If you have not had this conversation, it is important to be honest with the service user and explain your intention to pass on the information and your reasons for doing this.

2. It would be appropriate in this situation to seek support from your personal tutor who would be able to advise you on the possible ways you could respond. Alternatively, you may not feel comfortable managing this situation yourself and your personal tutor could approach the placement area on your behalf. Where your mentor's mental health is affecting their work and your learning, it would be advisable to do this immediately.

3. The HCA's practice in this scenario is questionable and may potentially be putting service users at risk. As a student nurse, you have a duty to report practice which could be unsafe, however this is often challenging to do. Many students are concerned about the consequences of making complaints and the impact this may have on how they are then treated in practice. If you have a trusting relationship with your mentor, it would be appropriate to report it to them and they would take action on your behalf. If you have concerns about doing this, you can also seek advice from your personal tutor who will guide you through the appropriate complaints procedure and support you during the process. While this is challenging, many students describe feeling a sense of pride in protecting service users and ensuring abuse does not go unchallenged.

Learning opportunities

1. It will be important for you and your mentor to discuss strategies which will ensure that you have the opportunity to meet your learning outcomes for that placement in light of the limited contact with service users. This could be achieved by doing some in-depth work with a small number of service users who are comfortable with your input. You could also arrange to spend time in a different clinical environment related to the work assertive outreach does. Time can also be spent reading policy and research relating to the service and considering how this applies to the service you are observing.

2. You are required to spend 40% of your time in placement with your mentor. If their role is preventing you from doing this, it would be important to raise this. If you are not comfortable doing this, then it would be appropriate to let your

personal tutor know so that they can query it on your behalf. While direct observation is one way of assessing your practice, your mentor will also consider reports from other members of the team, witness statements and your own reflective writing as evidence of your competence. Therefore, you do not need to work with your mentor continuously and there are benefits from working with other professionals such as observing different approaches and gaining other sources of feedback on your practice.

3. The paperwork associated with the nursing role is demanding and time-consuming, however there are ways of managing it in order to minimise the impact it has on contact with service users. You will often find that some nurses seem to spend more time doing paperwork than others. In this scenario, it is helpful to identify the nurses who you feel are managing to achieve this balance and ask their advice on how they accomplish this.

Further reading

Aston, L., Wakefield, J., McGowan, R., 2010. The student nurse guide to decision making in practice. Open University Press, Maidenhead.

Brooker, C., Waugh, A., 2007. Foundations of nursing practice: fundamentals of holistic care. Mosby, Edinburgh.

Burton, R., Ormrod, G., 2011. Nursing: transition to professional practice. Oxford University Press, Oxford.

Griffith, R., Tengnah, C., 2010. Law and professional issues in nursing, second ed. Learning Matters, Exeter.

Hindle, A., Coates, A., 2011. Nursing care of older people. Oxford University Press, Oxford.

Holland, K., Hogg, C., 2010. Cultural awareness in nursing and health care: an introductory text, second ed. Arnold, London.

Holland, K., Rees, C., 2010. Nursing: evidence-based practice skills. Oxford University Press, Oxford.

Levett-Jones, T., Bourgeois, S., 2009. The clinical placement, second ed. Baillière Tindall, Edinburgh.

Redfern, S., Ross, F.M., 2006. Nursing older people. Churchill Livingstone, Edinburgh.

Wrycraft, N., 2009. An introduction to mental health nursing. Open University Press, Maidenhead.

Websites

Royal College of Nursing: Mental Health Practice (*Student Life*: access to many resources if registered with the RCN and this journal): http://mentalhealthpractice. rcnpublishing.co.uk/resources/studentlife/ index.asp (accessed June 2011).

Appendix 1. Common acronyms used in mental health settings

AHP
Allied health professional

AMHP
Approved mental health practitioner

AO
Assertive outreach

BDI
Beck Depression Index

BME
Black and minority ethnic

BP
Blood pressure

BPD
Borderline personality disorder

CAMHS
Child and adolescent mental health

CBT
Cognitive behavioural therapy

CMHT
Community mental health team

CPA
Care Programme Approach

CPN
Community psychiatric nurse

CRHT
Crisis resolution and home treatment

CTO
Community treatment order

DBT
Dialectical behaviour therapy

DH
Department of Health

DPSD
Dangerous and severe personality disorder

ECT
Electroconvulsive therapy

EI
Early intervention

HONOS
Health of the Nation Outcome Scale

Appendix 1 Common acronyms used in mental health settings

IAPT
Increasing access to psychological therapies

LUNSERS
Liverpool University neuroleptic side effects rating scale

MHA
Mental Health Act

MSE
Mini-mental state examination

MVA
Managing violence and aggression

NICE
National Institute for Health and Clinical Excellence

NMC
Nursing and Midwifery Council

PD
Personality disorder

PICU
Psychiatric intensive care unit

PRN
Pro re nata (medication that is given when needed)

RC
Responsible clinician

SSRI
Selective serotonin reuptake inhibitor

STR
Support time and recovery (worker)

WRAP
Wellness recovery action plan

Appendix 2. Jargon buster

Accountability

A legal, ethical and moral responsibility to ensure that nursing practice is in the service user's best interests

Approved mental health professional (AMHP)

A mental health practitioner who has been trained to perform a pivotal role in assessing and deciding whether there are grounds to detain a person who is experiencing mental health problems without their consent

Autonomous

The ethical right to make an informed and free decision

Clinical supervision

A facilitated discussion which aims to encourage the practitioner to reflect and learn from their clinical experiences

Collaboration

Working together towards a common goal

Compliant

Following a recommended course of action or treatment

Concordant

Having involvement in decision-making processes

Confidentiality

A legal and professional responsibility to ensure information regarding service users is only available to those who are authorised to have access

Consent

Giving approval of a decision or action after consideration

Defensive practice

Practice which is primarily concerned with preventing possible malpractice legal action as opposed to the service users' best interests

Delusion

A belief that is held by a person despite a lack of evidence to support its truth

Direct payments

Local council payments for people who have been assessed as needing help from social services, and who would like to arrange and pay for their own care and support services instead of receiving them directly from the local council

Discrimination

Excluding or restricting members of one group from opportunities that are available to others

Dual diagnosis

People who have a substance misuse problem and a mental health problem

Expressed emotion

The level of feeling displayed in families or teams towards a person with mental health problems

Hallucination

An unusual perception which is there when we are awake and has qualities of real perceptions

Human rights

The freedoms that all humans are entailed to

Informal service user (patient)

A person who is an in-patient in a 24-hour care setting but has not been legally detained against their will

Mania

The presence of extremely high energy levels and elevated mood

Mental Capacity Act

Primarily concerned with providing a legal framework for acting and making decisions on behalf of adults who lack the ability to make particular decisions for themselves

Mental Health Act

Primarily concerned with providing a legal framework to allow people to be detained in hospital against their will for assessment and treatment of mental health problems (also known as sectioning)

Multidisciplinary

Involvement of a number of professional groups with the aim of providing an integrated approach to care

Nearest relative

A close relative who the AMHP has identified from a hierarchy defined in the Mental Health Act. The nearest relative has the right to request an assessment for their relative to be detained in hospital and apply for their relative to be discharged from a Section which has been enforced

Neurotransmitters

Chemicals which pass messages from a neuron to a target cell

Personal budgets

An allocation of funding given to service users after an assessment which should be sufficient to meet their assessed needs. Users can either take their personal budget as a direct payment, or, while still choosing how their care needs are met and by whom, leave councils with the responsibility to commission the services

Prejudice

An assumption made about someone without having sufficient or accurate knowledge to make a judgement

PRN medication

Medication which is given when needed or when a specific situation arises

Prodromal symptom

An early sign which can indicate the start of an illness before specific symptoms relating to that illness occur

Psychiatry

The medical specialty focused on the assessment and treatment of mental disorder

Psychoeducation

Information shared with the service user and their family about the possible cause, nature and treatment of mental health problems

Psychosis/psychotic

A medical term used to describe people who are experiencing voices, unusual perceptions or expressing unusual beliefs

Psychotropic medication

Drugs which act on the central nervous system to alter brain function resulting in changes in perception, mood, consciousness, thoughts and behaviour

Reflection

The self-observation of personal thoughts, behaviours and influence on others

Relapse signature

The unique signs that indicate a person's level of distress is increasing

Relapse drill

The pre-agreed actions which should be taken during periods of increased distress to reduce the likelihood of relapse or the disruption caused by relapse

Responsible clinician (RC)

The approved clinician with overall responsibility for the service user's case

Sectioning

Unofficial term for use of the Mental Health Act to detain a person in hospital against their will

Social exclusion

The multiple effects of discrimination including loss of roles, relationships and access to community and financial resources

Social inclusion

Regaining hope, a sense of personal control and access to opportunities

STAT dose

A single dose of medication which is given immediately

Statutory/public sector

Services which are provided by the government and funded by taxes

Voluntary/independent sector

Services which are provided by charities or self-regulated organisations. These services may be partly funded by the government through the provision of grant schemes. Alternatively, they may be paid for by the individual accessing the service or through charitable donations

Index

Page numbers ending in 'b', 'f' and 't' refer to Boxes, Figures and Tables respectively

Index

Index

Index

Index

Index

Printed in the United States
By Bookmasters